Obesity

Edited by Hülya Çakmur

Published in London, United Kingdom

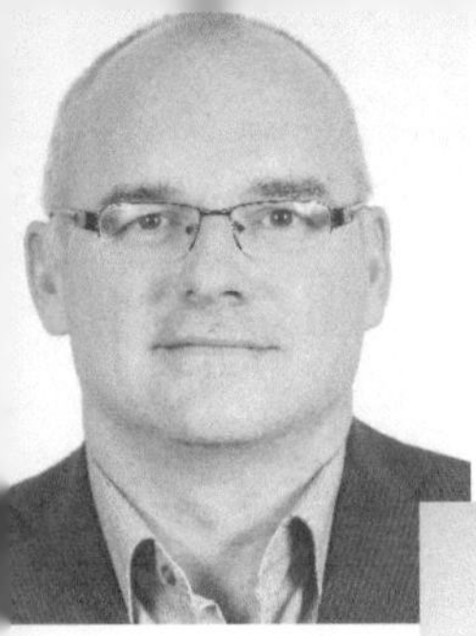
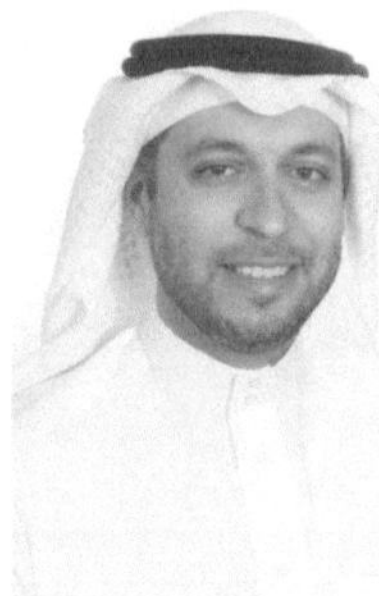
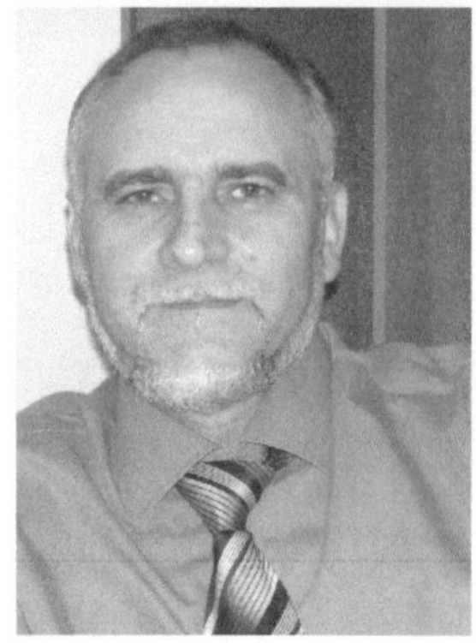
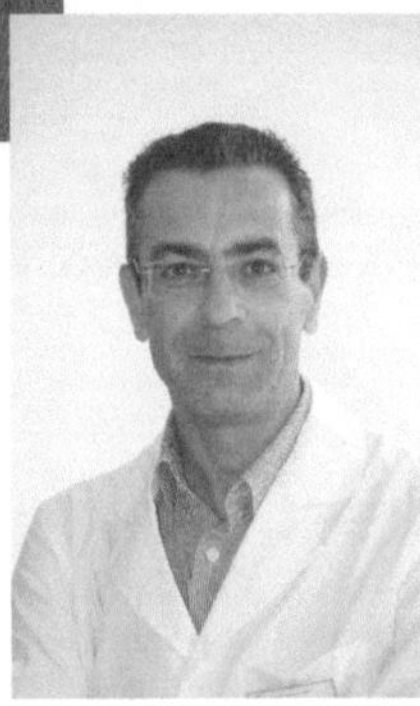
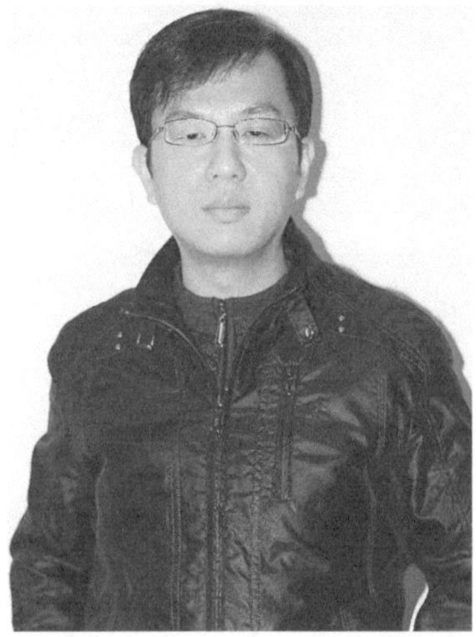
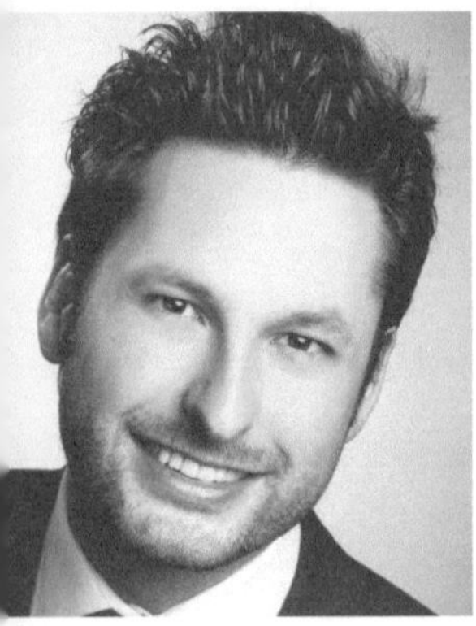
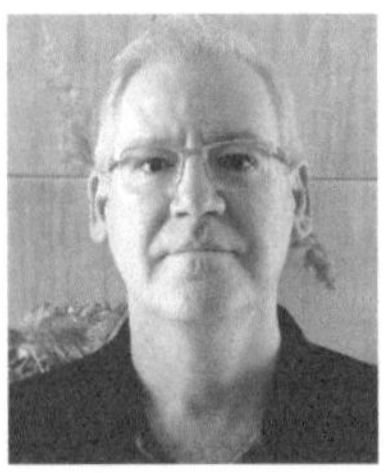

IntechOpen

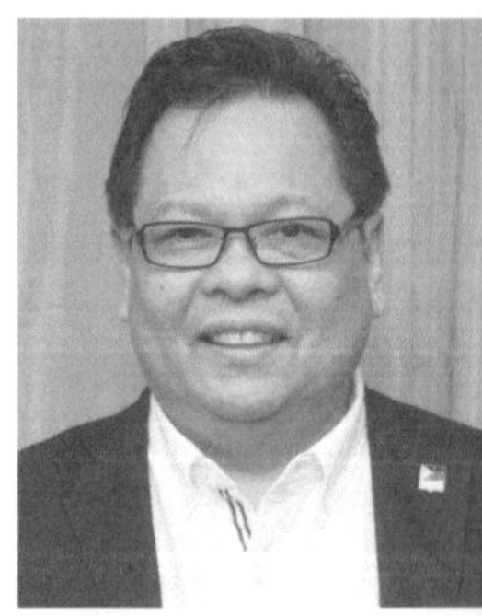
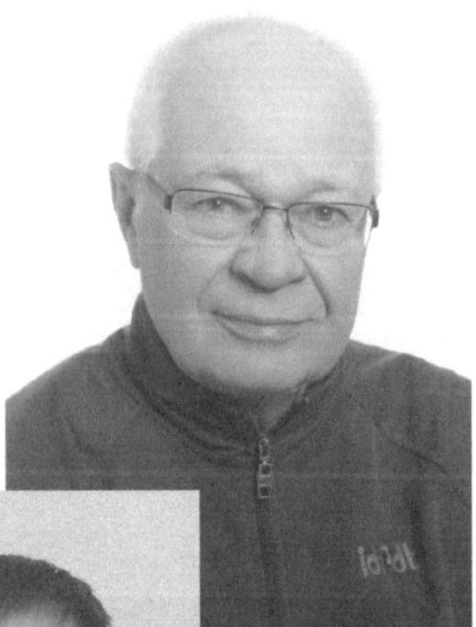
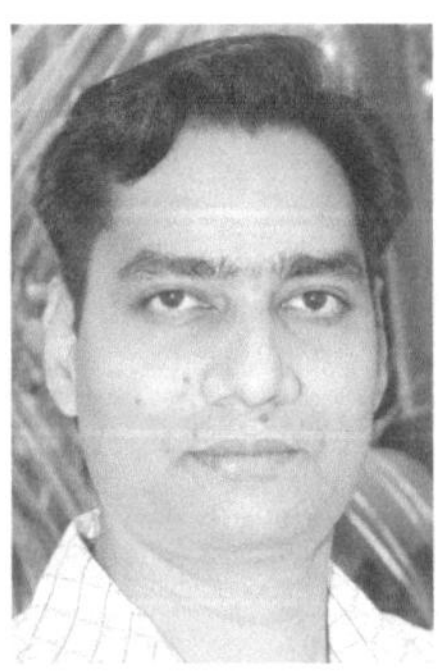
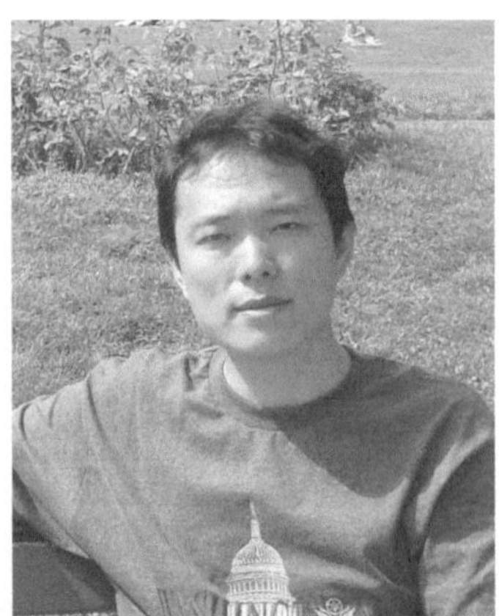
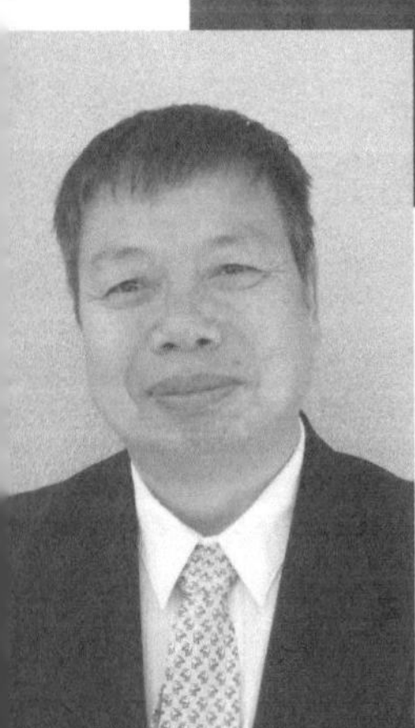
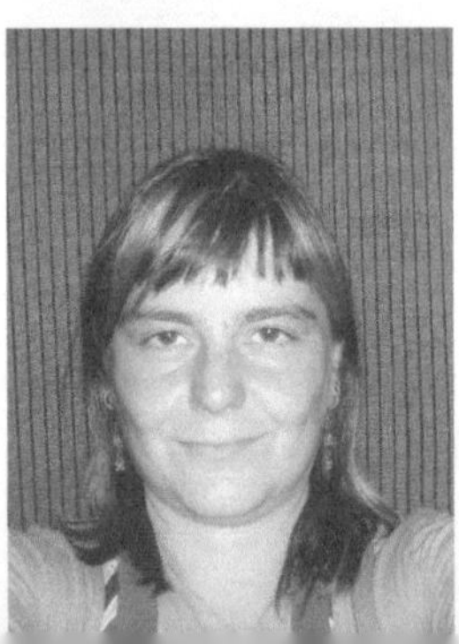

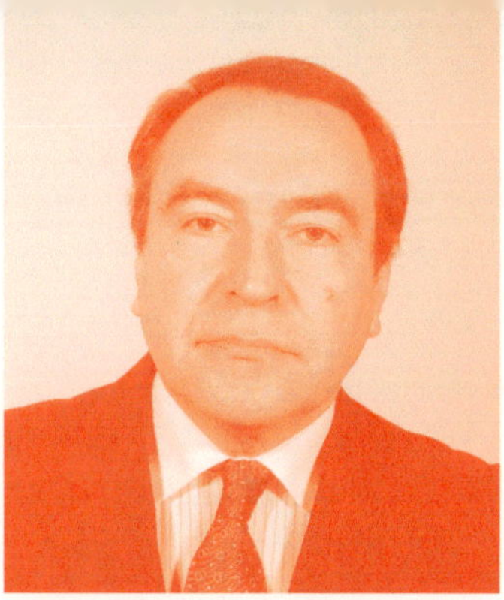
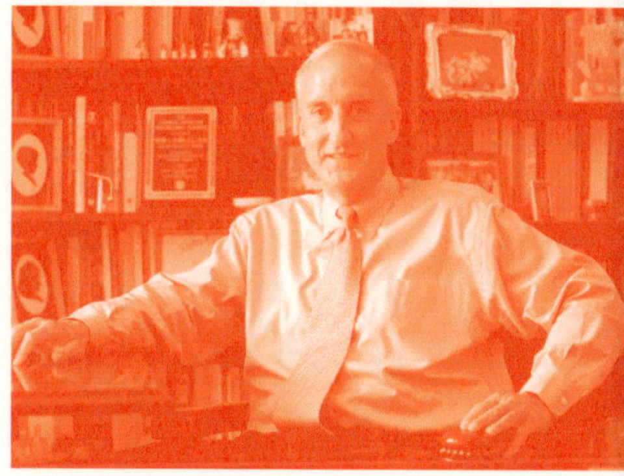
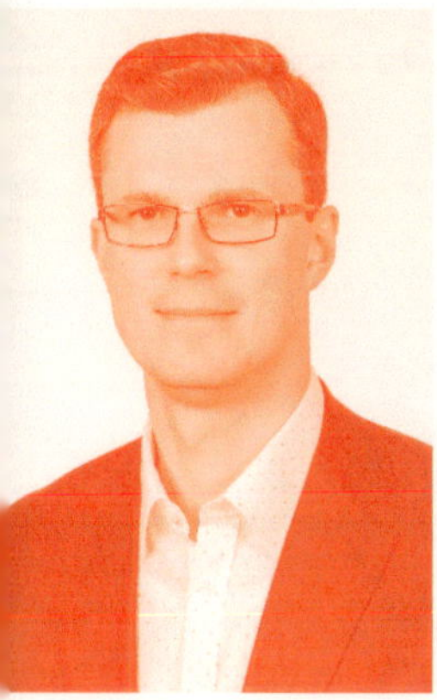
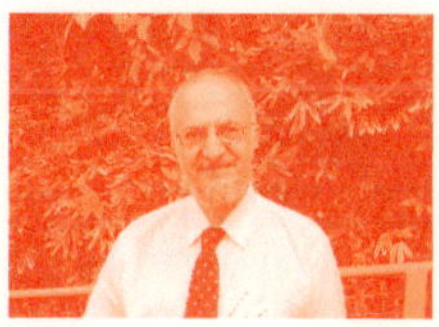
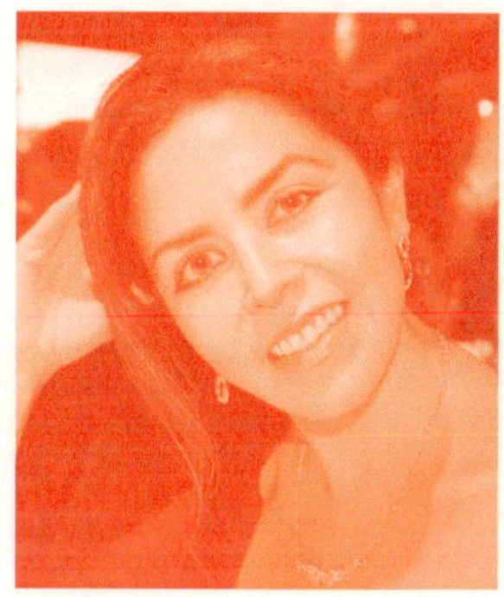

Supporting open minds since 2005

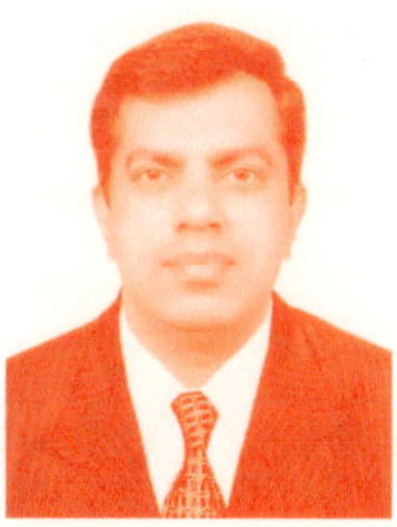
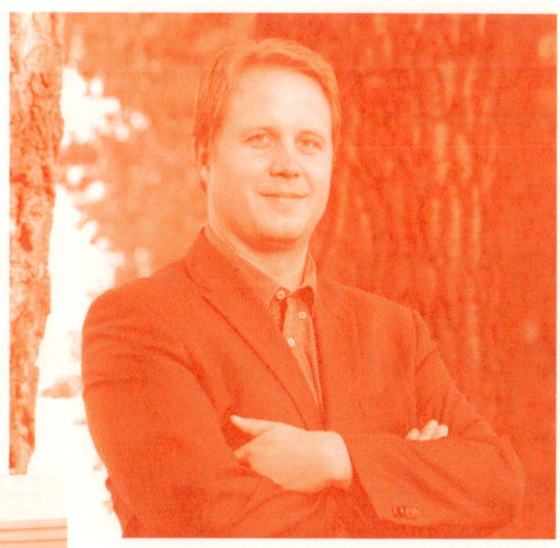
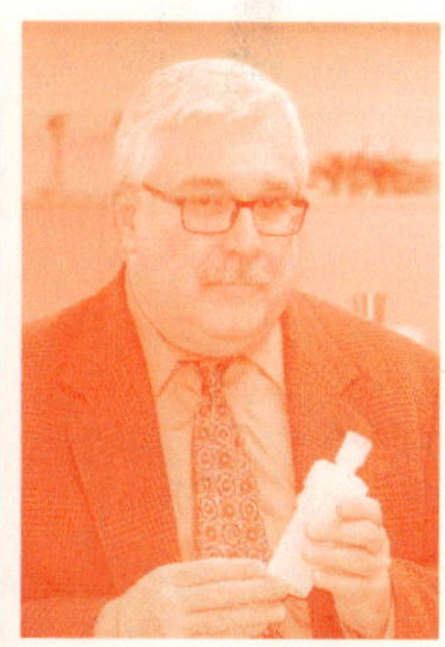
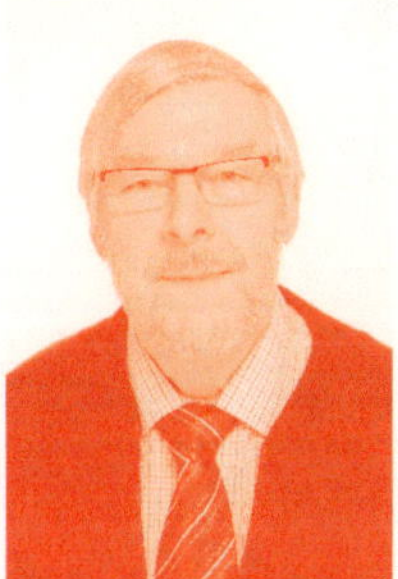
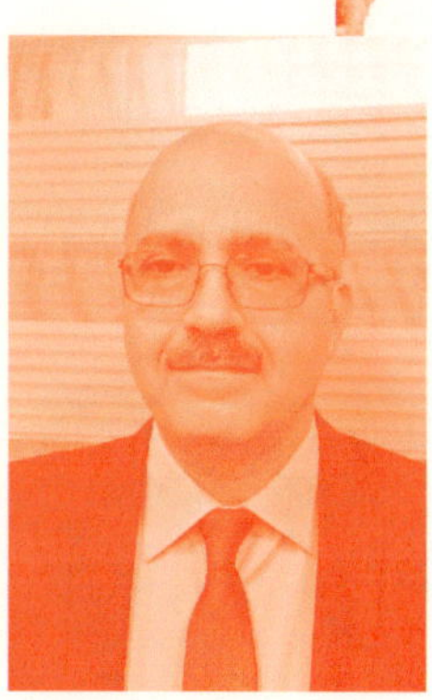
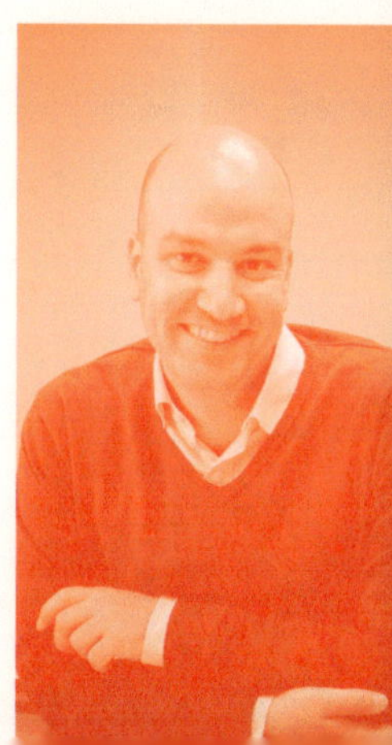
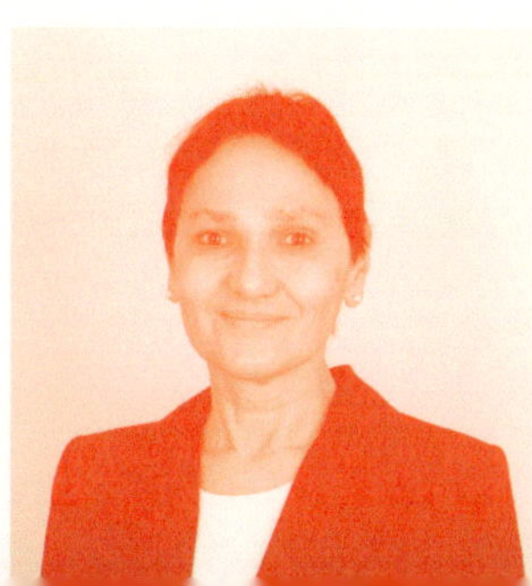

Obesity
http://dx.doi.org/10.5772/intechopen.73774
Edited by Hülya Çakmur

Contributors
Kathleen DeCicco-Skinner, Nicole Bonan, Roger Hart, Tamara Hunter, Hülya Çakmur, Tülay Diken Diken Allahverdi, J. Aureliano Robles-De Anda, Gustavo Ignacio Diaz-Rubio, Fernanda Isadora Corona Meraz, Perla-Monserrat Madrigal-Ruiz, Jorge Castro-Albarran, Rosa Elena Navarro Hernandez

First published in London, United Kingdom, 2020 by IntechOpen
IntechOpen is the global imprint of INTECHOPEN LIMITED, registered in England and Wales, registration number: 11086078, 7th floor, 10 Lower Thames Street, London, EC3R 6AF, United Kingdom
Printed in Croatia

British Library Cataloguing-in-Publication Data
A catalogue record for this book is available from the British Library

Additional hard and PDF copies can be obtained from orders@intechopen.com

Obesity
Edited by Hülya Çakmur
p. cm.
Print ISBN 978-1-78985-494-7
Online ISBN 978-1-78985-852-5
eBook (PDF) ISBN 978-1-78985-885-3

Meet the editor

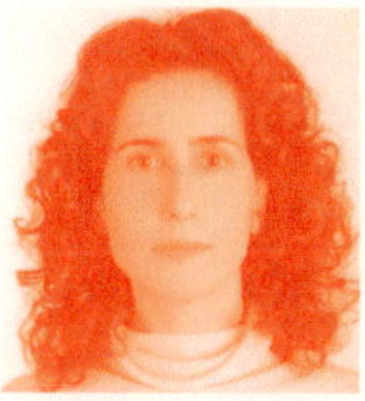

Hülya Çakmur graduated from medical school at Atatürk University in Turkey. She completed her residency training in family medicine at Trakya University. She has 20 years of practice experience as a specialist in family medicine, including 8 years of experience in public health as a PhD-prepared professional. She completed her PhD in Public Health at Dokuz Eylül University. She studied sleep medicine at UPMC in the United States, attended narrative medicine education at STU in Canada, and studied voluntarily in geriatrics. She has published several studies in the field of elderly health and is an active member of the Turkish Medical Association and European Academy of Teachers in General Practice/Family Medicine. She has seven years of teaching experience as an associate professor at the University of Kafkas and is the director of the Department of Family Medicine. She has published more than 25 papers in reputed journals.

Contents

Preface

Why is humanity in general becoming obese but some parts of the world are suffering from starvation? Ironically, this problem of socioeconomic disparity is becoming increasingly prevalent in almost every continent. Unfortunately, it is not an intended situation, such as health problems caused by being underweight. Obesity could be defined as a multifactorial and heterogeneous disease.
Higher morbidity and mortality rates are associated with obesity. Excessive fat accumulation is seen as the etiological reason for almost all chronic diseases. Obesity threatens human health and reduces life expectancy. Genetic, biological, environmental, and behavioral factors (binge eating/drinking, laziness, lack of willpower, insufficient sleep, sedentary lifestyle, and self-indulgence) are blamed for the pathogenesis of obesity. Environmental factors (low socioeconomic status, lack of education, cultural reasons, and environmental pollution), family lifestyle, eating habits, and inactivity also play important roles in obesity. When biological factors (disability, gut microbiota, comorbidities, and prenatal, neural, and endocrine conditions) and genetics interact with behavioral and/or environmental factors, the result is obesity. Oxidative damage is the main underlying mechanism of obesity-related diseases. As the prevalence of obesity increases, morbidity and mortality from obesity-related diseases also increase. In addition, obesity-related health problems increase treatment costs and lead to financial and labor losses in society. Population-based, preventive, and sustainable public health approaches are necessary to combat obesity. Obesity is preventable, and healthcare professionals have an important role to play in preventing this problem. Healthcare policy objectives must be centered on improving life expectancy and quality of life for humanity all over the world. Healthy and supportive environments are indispensable factors for preventing obesity, in addition to education. However, the fundamental issue is the processed food industry.

Hülya Çakmur
Kafkas University,
Turkey

Chapter 1

Introductory Chapter: Unbearable Burden of the Diseases - Obesity

Hülya Çakmur

1. Obesity definition measurement and classification

Obesity and overweight are commonly accepted as immoderate fat accumulation in human body that increases the risk of almost every disease [1, 2]. Excessive fat accumulation is usually measured by body mass index (BMI), which is calculated with the weight and height proportions (weight relative to square of the height-w/h^2) [3]. A reliable measurement of the fat accumulation requires elaborated tool such as magnetic resonance imaging (bio-electrical impedance). Because of the Bio-electrical Impedance Analysis is not widely available, BMI is accepted population-based definition and classification tool of obesity and overweight. Twenty percent and above fat accumulation in human body is accepted as normal [3]. If the level exceeds this limit (according to standard age, height, and weight tables), it is defined as overweight and obesity [3, 4]. BMI is a commonly used indicator of obesity and it classifies as follows (kg/m^2): <18.5 for underweight, 18.5–24.9 for normal weight, 25–29.9 for overweight, and ≥30 for obese [4]. Sometimes, BMI shows normal limits even in the presence of abdominal (central) obesity. So the central obesity, which is a kind of more risky obesity, could be hidden [4, 5]. It has been reported that almost half of the children and adults with excess body fat are defined as nonobese according to BMI [6, 7]. Underestimates of obesity prevalence could lead to less attention to problems and inadequate prevention and combat. Bioelectrical impedance uses tetra-polar measurements by touch electrodes and the measurements include broad spectrum from visceral fat mass to subcutaneous fat mass and body fat over [8]. Thus, misinterpretation of obesity and overweight can be prevented. Maximum attention is required to correct the evaluation of adipose tissue dissemination and measurements. Health care professionals must be aware of hidden obesity.

2. Obesity pathogenesis

The most widely accepted opinion about obesity pathogenesis is that it is the result of balance mechanism between energy intake and expenditure. Recent investigation indicates that obesity pathogenesis is more complex than just an energy imbalance. The mechanism of energy intake and expenditure is a homeostatic process [9, 10–12]. This balance mechanism regulates body weight in "normal" limits. Earlier, obesity was thought just as an extreme calorie consumption than what the body needs. But researches and inventions in medicine show that the mechanism and etiology of obesity are not so simple. Reported studies showed that obesity pathogenesis is not only based on excess energy expenditure but also on the body's urge to fix and maintain the weight at an augmented value [9, 11, 13–15]. This process would explain why obesity does not respond to long-lasting diet and exercise program or why there is no permanent reduction in weight even if there is a response [12].

The main issue is to understand that why human body keep adipose tissue. Extreme fat accumulation actually is a biological defense mechanism of the adipose tissue [13]. Adipose tissue is a storage and endocrine organ needed for energy homeostasis. It is well known that the regulation of energy homeostasis depends on the adipose tissue. Recently, studies revealed that especially the visceral compartment of the adipose tissue not only simply deposits energy but also plays an active role in endocrine metabolism and immune system [12, 14, 16]. To comprehend pathogenesis of obesity needs to understand how adipose tissue works. Adipose tissue (composed of adipocytes-fat cells) has important roles in glucose homeostasis, immune responses, hormonal regulation, and reproductive functions. Fat cells (adipocytes) are derived from mesenchymal stem cells. Preadipocytes become adipocytes through the cell differentiation process called adipogenesis. [11, 13, 16]. It has been shown that adipocytes secrete biologically active molecules called adipocytokines. Some of these are tumor necrosis factor-α (TNF-α), adiponectin, visfatin, omentin, cytokines, resistin, retinol-binding protein 4, and leptin. In case of excessive fat accumulation, pro-inflammatory cytokines such as tumor necrosis factor-alpha, interleukin (IL)-1β, and IL-6 are released. TNF-α is a main cytokine in the inflammatory response. It is well known that the serum TNF-α levels are increased in obesity and decreased in case of weight loss. Because of an active interaction of adipocytokines, obesity is regarded as a chronic inflammation in the human body. It is clearly known that the adipose tissue expands so that the circulating inflammation-related adipocytokines increase. Excessive fat accumulation continually increased oxidative stress (OS) [16–18]. OS leads to inflammatory reaction by triggering acute-phase response. Adipose tissue contains white and brown adipocytes. The white adipose tissue (WAT) is chiefly responsible for fat accumulation. WAT stores energy as triglycerides [11]. The brown adipose tissue (BAT) is an important energy source for the human body. It is responsible for the thermogenic activity. There is plenty of brown adipose tissue during infancy to adolescent surrounding the heart and large vessels. It has been shown that BAT decreases as humans mature. A mature human body has few brown adipose tissues as scattered cells within white fat pads. The brown adipocytes are multilocular and contain less lipid. [19]. Recently, it has been shown that the brown adipose tissue could be increased with the catecholamine discharge. To living in cold area increase brown adipose tissue. This specificity could be used effectively for combating obesity. Biologically, humans are prone to conserve body fat as a defense mechanism in case of starvation and famine. The theory of "thrifty gene" claimed that human genes were predisposed to accumulate adipose tissue for use in case of energy requirement [1, 11, 19]. This mechanism was a key factor for survival once. Over time, the problem of finding food disappeared. However, human biology and physiology failed to adapt to this quick change. Humans' evolutionary biology remained slow in the face of fast transformation of environmental conditions (easily reachable abundant foods). Human genes which is predisposed to excessive weight gain pursued their tasks in present of the today's world. Genes are not the only factors that lead to obesity. Excessive fat accumulation is a multifactorial disorder. First of all, it is a disorder of the energy homeostasis system [10–13]. Still, the fundamental reason that leads to obesity is energy imbalance between energy intake and expenditure. Examining all these factors comprehensively could provide an understanding of the pathogenesis of obesity. The main factors in the pathogenesis of obesity were claimed to be behavioral, biological, environmental, and molecular [1, 12]. All these factors contribute to fat accumulation on a different level. Generally, personal traits (binge eating-drinking, laziness, lack of will power, insufficient sleep, sedentary life style, and self-indulgence) were accused as behavioral factors that lead to excess weight gain [9, 10]. Biological factors include disability, gut microbiota, comorbidity, and prenatal, neural, and endocrine conditions besides genetics. Environmental factors that lead to obesity are socioeconomic status, cultural reasons, and environmental pollutions. On a molecular level, the pathogenesis of obesity is based on the impairment of electron transport chain. Low education and socioeconomic level, family lifestyle, eating habits, and inactivity play important roles in obesity [1–3, 9, 10]. When the interaction of biological factors with behavioral and/or environmental factors is abundant, excessive fat accumulation is inevitable. Until now, the pathogenesis of obesity is not clarified entirely, but it is believed to be a disorder with multiple causes. The current opinion is that obesity is a multifactorial and heterogeneous disease that leads to adverse cellular and metabolic effects.

3. How obesity causes diseases

It is well known that obesity and overweight are major risk factors for many acute and chronic diseases from metabolic and mental to cancer [20–23]. There is no doubt that obesity is a disease of its own, but it is also the main cause of various diseases in human body. The underlying mechanisms of obesity-related diseases are not well understood, but many evidences have pointed to cellular oxidative stress, following oxidative damage [16–18]. The expansion of the adipose tissue especially increases the visceral fat accumulation. Excessive energy mainly deposit in adipose tissue as triglyceride. It has been shown that visceral fat accumulation leads to many chronic diseases. Blood glucose and lipids are continually high in obesity. Increased levels of glucose and lipids in circulation lead to excessive energy substrates in adipose tissue, which increase the production of reactive oxygen species (ROS) [1, 12, 16–18]. It is well known that ROS is related to chronic inflammation in the human body. Excessive production of ROS can lead to cellular damage and cellular dysfunction by disrupting the structures of proteins, lipids, and nucleic acids. Obesity is a chronic systemic inflammation of the adipose tissue. Long-lasting obesity eventually activates the innate immune system in adipose tissue. Excessive fat accumulation continually increases oxidative stress (OS), which leads to inflammatory reaction by triggering acute-phase response. OS-activated immune cells generate free radicals. Adipokines also induce the production of reactive oxygen species in the same way. The inflammation of adipose tissue plays a critical role in obesity-related diseases. Intensive and permanent oxidative stress damages cellular structures. Additionally, in case of insufficient antioxidant capacity, obesity-related complications easily emerge [1, 12, 16–18]. Thus obesity led to the cardiovascular, gastrointestinal, genitourinary, metabolic/endocrine, musculoskeletal/orthopedic, neurological and central nervous, obstetric and perinatal, skin, psychological, respiratory/pulmonary, and reproductive systems [1–3]. Studies to understand the pathogenesis of obesity and obesity-related diseases are continuing rapidly. Fully comprehending the molecular mechanisms of obesity and obesity-related diseases would lead to the discovery of new therapies and preventive methods.

4. Obesity prevalence

Obesity was not common until the twentieth century. The World Health Organization (WHO) formally accepted obesity as a global epidemic in 1997 [2]. Obesity prevalence steadily increased in the following years. The prevalence of obesity doubled in the last 40 years. Almost 50% of the adults are overweight and obese in many countries. WHO has reported obesity prevalence (2015) in some countries such as: Cook Island: 89%, Qatar: 42%, UAE: 37%, Saudi Arabia: 34%, Turkey: 29%,

Egypt: 28%, Australia: 28%, UK: 28%, France: 23%, Italy: 21%, Sweden: 20%, Germany: 20%, Brazil: 20%, and Japan: 3%. [2, 3, 24]. The worst is that obesity affects children all around the world. It has been reported that a quarter of children around the world are obese. The prevalence of obesity is especially high in industrialized countries, but it is also dramatically increasing in developing countries. Obesity prevalence is higher in low-income and low-educated people and the rate of obesity increases with age. Female gender is a risk factor for obesity especially in developing countries. [2, 3, 7, 24].

5. Combating obesity

As the prevalence of obesity increases, the morbidity and mortality from obesity-related diseases (mainly cardiovascular diseases, diabetes, and various cancers) also increase [9, 24–26]. Obesity and obesity-related morbidities require careful clinical assessment. Obesity-related health problems also increase the treatment cost and lead to financial and labor loss in society [27]. As an effective strategy to combating obesity, population-based, preventive, and sustainable public health approaches are necessary. Specialized public health strategies for the risk groups such as children, adolescent, low-educated, and disabled people are also important to reduce and prevent obesity. Obesity is preventable and health care professionals have an important role in preventing it. Aim of the health care policies is to increase the life expectancy and more qualified life span for human beings all over the world. Healthy and supportive environments are indispensable to combat obesity [28, 29]. Education is the most important step for challenging obesity. The training program should be implemented at every opportunity to effect people's choices, by making basic healthy life-style choices (i.e., regular physical activity, healthier foods, etc.). Lifestyle factors and personal responsibility are efficient to some degree to decrease the prevalence of obesity. However, more effective measures are required to cope with an epidemic of obesity at the societal level. Parents must be enlightened about obesity to prevent childhood obesity. Obese children mostly become obese adults. Healthier food choices are provided in school. Obesity awareness must be increased by educative programs (such as school-based education about nutrition and dietary guidelines) [30, 31]. The fundamental issue is to produce healthier and unprocessed foods for the growing world population. Food marketing and pricing policies should be changed in favor of the people, not the industry.

6. Key points

- Obesity could be defined as a multifactorial and heterogeneous disease.
- Obesity is a chronic systemic inflammation of the adipose tissue.
- Adipose tissue is a storage and endocrine organ needed for energy homeostasis.
- Fat accumulation actually is a biological defense mechanism of the adipose tissue.
- Excessive fat accumulation continually increases oxidative stress.
- The underlying mechanisms of obesity-related diseases are associated with the oxidative damage.

- The main factors in the pathogenesis of obesity are claimed to be genetic, biological, behavioral, environmental, and molecular.
- Obesity is a major risk factor for several diseases from metabolic and mental to cancer.
- Obesity reduces life expectancy and increases the risk of mortality.
- Almost 50% of adults are overweight and obese in many countries.
- A quarter of children around the world are obese and obese children mostly become obese adults.
- BMI is a commonly used indicator for obesity, but central obesity could be hidden.
- Obesity-related health problems also increase the treatment cost and lead to financial and labor loss in society.
- The prevalence of obesity is higher in low-income and low-educated people and the rate of obesity increases with age. Female gender is a risk factor for obesity especially in developing countries.
- Obesity is preventable. Population-based, preventive, and sustainable public health approaches are necessary to combat an epidemic of obesity.

Author details

Hülya Çakmur
Kafkas University, Turkey

*Address all correspondence to: hulyacakmur@gmail.com

References

[1] Haslam DW, James WP. Obesity. Lancet. 2005;**366**:1197-1209. DOI: 10.1111/j.1467-789X.2009.00708

[2] WHO. Global Strategy on Diet, Physical Activity and Health Solarex. [Internet]. 2015. Available from: http://www.who.int/features/factfiles/obesity/en/ [Accessed: 12-11-2018]

[3] World Health Organization Technical Report Series 854. Physical Status: The Use and Interpretation of Anthropometry. Geneva 1995. pp. 312-17. [Internet]. Avaliable from: http://www.euro.who.int/data/assets/pdf_file/0011/199532/Health2020-Long.pdf/0010/74746/E90711.pdf. [Accessed: 12-10-2018]

[4] Croghan IT, Phelan SM, Bradley DP, Bauer KW, Seung-Young-Han, Bradley SM, et al. Needs assessment for weight management: The learning health system network experience. Mayo Clinic Proceedings: Innovations, Quality & Outcomes. 2018;**2**(4):324-335. DOI: 10.1016/j.mayocpiqo.2018.08.001

[5] Barberio AM, Alareeki A, Viner B, Pader J, Vena JE, Arora P, et al. Central body fatness is a stronger predictor of cancer risk than overall body size. Nature Communications. 2019;**10**(1):383. DOI: 10.1038/s41467-018-08159-w

[6] Javed A, Jumean M, Murad MH. Diagnostic performance of body mass index to identify obesity as defined by body adiposity in children and adolescents: A systematic review and meta-analysis. Pediatric Obesity. 2015;**10**:234-244

[7] Reilly JJ, Kelly J, Wilson DC. Accuracy of simple clinical and epidemiological definitions of childhood obesity: Systematic review and evidence appraisal. Obesity Reviews. 2010;**11**:645-655

[8] Metcalf B, Rabkin RA, Rabkin JM, Metcalf LJ, Lehman-Becker LB. Weight loss composition: The effects of exercise following obesity surgery as measured by bioelectrical impedance analysis. Obesity Surgery. 2005;**15**(2):183-186

[9] Mathus-Vliegen EMH, Basdevant A, Finer N, Hainer V, Hauner H, Micic D, et al. Prevalence, pathophysiology, health consequences and treatment options of obesity in the elderly: A guideline. Obesity Facts. 2012;**5**: 460-483. DOI: 10.1159/000341193

[10] Wolin KY, Petrelli JM. Obesity. Santa Barbara, CA: Greenwood Press; 2009. ISBN 10: 0313352763/ISBN 13: 9780313352768

[11] Rosen ED, Spiegelman BM. Adipocytes as regulators of energy balance and glucose homeostasis. Nature. 2006;**444**:847-853. DOI: 10.1038/nature05483

[12] Trayhurn P. The biology of obesity. The Proceedings of the Nutrition Society. 2005;**64**(1):31-38

[13] Lefterova MI, Lazar MA. New developments in adipogenesis. Trends in Endocrinology and Metabolism. 2009;**20**:107-114. DOI: 10.1016/j.tem.2008.11.005

[14] Blaszczak AM, Jalilvand A, Liu J, Wright VP, Suzo A, Needleman B, et al. Human visceral adipose tissue macrophages are not adequately defined by standard methods of characterization. Journal Diabetes Research. 2019:8124563. DOI: 10.1155/2019/8124563

[15] Sharon MF. Obesity: Risk factors, complications, and strategies for sustainable longterm weight management. Journal of the American Association of Nurse Practitioners. 2017;**29**(Suppl 1):3-14

[16] Marseglia L, Manti S, D'Angelo G, Nicotera A, Parisi E, Di Rosa G, et al. Oxidative stress in obesity: A critical component in human diseases. International Journal of Molecular Sciences. 2015;**16**(1):378-400

[17] Kern L, Mittenbühler MJ, Vesting AJ, Ostermann AL, Wunderlich CM, Wunderlich FT. Obesity-induced TNFα and IL-6 signaling: The missing link between obesity and inflammation-driven liver and colorectal cancers. Cancers (Basel). 2018;**11**(1). pii: E24. DOI: 10.3390/ cancers11010024

[18] Furukawa S, Fujita T, Shimabukuro M, Iwaki M, Yamada Y, Nakajima Y, et al. Increased oxidative stress in obesity and its impact on metabolic syndrome. The Journal of Clinical Investigation. 2004;**114**(12):1752-1761. DOI: 10.1172/JCI200421625

[19] Sellayah D. The impact of early human migration on Brown adipose TissueEvolution and its relevance to the modern obesity pandemic. Journal of the Endocrine Society. 2018;**3**(2): 372-386. DOI: 10.1210/js.2018-00363

[20] Landsberg L, Aronne LJ, Beilin LJ, Burke V, Igel LI, Lloyd-Jones D, et al. Obesity related hypertension: Pathogenesis, cardiovascular risk, and treatment-a position paper of the Obesity Society and the American Society of Hypertension. Obesity. 2013;(1):8-24. DOI: 10.1002/oby.20181

[21] Çakmur H, Ardıç S. Investıgatıon of obesıty and depressıon ın a sample of Turkısh elderly adults. Turkish Journal of Geriatrics. 2015;**2**:115-122

[22] Roberts DL, Dive C, Renehan AG. Biological mechanisms linking obesity and cancer risk: New perspectives. Annual Review of Medicine. 2010;**61**:301-316. DOI: 10.1146/annurev.med.080708.082713

[23] Xu YXZ, Mishra S. Obesity-linked cancers: Current knowledge, challenges and limitations in mechanistic studies and rodent models. Cancers (Basel) 2018;**18**(12):10. pii: E523. DOI: 10.3390/ cancers10120523

[24] Berghöfer A, Pischon T, Reinhold T, Apovian CM, Sharma AM, Willich SN. Obesity prevalence from a European perspective: A systematic review. BMC Public Health. 2008;**8**:200. DOI: 10.1186/1471-2458-8-200

[25] Roberto CA, Swinburn B, Hawkes C, Huang TT, Costa SA, Ashe M, et al. Patchy progress on obesity prevention: Emerging examples, entrenched barriers, and new thinking. Lancet. 2015;**385**(9985):2400-2409. DOI: 10.1016/S0140-6736(14)61744-X

[26] Montgomery MK, De Nardo W, Watt MJ. Impact of lipotoxicity on tissue "cross talk" and metabolic regulation. Physiology (Bethesda, Md.). 2019;**34**(2):134-149. DOI: 10.1152/ physiol.00037.2018

[27] Withrow DA, Alter D. The economic burden of obesity worldwide: A systematic review of the direct costs of obesity. Obesity Reviews. 2011;**12**:131-141. DOI: 10.1111/j.1467-789X. 2009.00712

[28] LeBlanc-Morales N. Culinary medicine: Patient education for therapeutic lifestyle changes. Critical Care Nursing Clinics of North America. 2019;**31**(1):109-123. DOI: 10.1016/j. cnc.2018.11.009. Epub 2018 Dec 24

[29] Volger S, Rigassio Radler D, Rothpletz-Puglia P. Early childhood obesity prevention efforts through a life course health development perspective: A scoping review. PLoS One. 2018;**13**(12):e0209787. DOI: 10.1371/ journal.pone.0209787

[30] Bramante CT, Thornton RLJ, Bennett WL, Zhang A, Wilson RF, Bass EB, et al. Systematic review of natural experiments for childhood

obesity prevention and control. American Journal of Preventive Medicine. 2019;**56**(1):147-158. DOI: 10.1016/j.amepre.2018.08.023

[31] Stoner L, Beets MW, Brazendale K, Moore JB, Weaver RG. Exercise dose and weight loss in adolescents with overweight-obesity: A meta-regression. Sports Medicine. 2019;**49**(1):83-94. DOI: 10.1007/s40279-018-01040-2

Chapter 2

Adipose Tissue in Health and Disease

Fernanda-Isadora Corona-Meraz,
Jesus-Aureliano Robles-De Anda,
Perla-Monserrat Madrigal-Ruiz, Gustavo-Ignacio Díaz-Rubio,
Jorge Castro-Albarrán and Rosa-Elena Navarro-Hernández

Abstract

Obesity, being an epidemy these days, is the trigger of metabolic disturbances such as cardiovascular disease, type 2 diabetes, and insulin resistance. Defined as an increase in fat storage, adipose tissue has been put under the spotlight as the culprit of these conditions, as it is composed not only by adipocytes but of any immune system cell and a singular extracellular matrix. Its behavior under acute and chronic hypercaloric states is quite different; persistent hypertrophy in the latter creates hypoxia, resulting in the release of reactive oxygen species and proinflammatory cytokines that impact on the immune response type of the resident leucocytes, mainly macrophages. Hypertrophy over hyperplasia, adipose tissue macrophages-M1 phenotype polarization, and the adipokines/myokines profile are thought to be regulated by foreign microRNAs, delivered from surrounding or distant cells by exosomes through the bloodstream. In this chapter, we focus on adipose tissue immunometabolism and how obesity causes the chronic inflammatory state, and, subsequently, this stablishes a pathologic adiposity, characterized by dyslipidemia and insulin resistance (IR).

Keywords: obesity, adipose tissue, adipose tissue macrophages-M1 phenotype, exosomes, microRNAs, insulin resistance, pathologic adiposity

1. Introduction

Novel findings on the immune-regulatory processes and metabolic mechanisms may open new avenues in the complex diseases as well as obesity; research on basic and clinical advances in immunometabolism has evolved rapidly during the past years, and the emergence of new tools for the detection and characterization of regulation of inflammation in systemic inflammatory diseases with metabolic comorbidity may play an imperative role.

Interplay in regulation of inflammation and metabolic risk factors are a complex cluster. The inflammatory condition associated with adipose tissue represents a triggering factor in the etiology of the obesity pathological-mechanism and mainly contributes to the related disease outcomes.

The purpose of this chapter is to address recent findings in metabolic, molecular biology, function, and pathology of the immune response to inflammation on the role of the immunometabolism in obesity. That containing significant new findings in the field, presenting the state of the art findings, will offer the new insights into interplay in the regulation of inflammation, especially in the tools of the comorbidity, in order to know their mechanisms by metabolic and immune response that cause disease.

2. Healthy adipose tissue

2.1 Morphology and cellular biology

Adipose tissue (AT) is a type of specialized connective tissue, and as such, it consists of two main components: a cellular population and a specialized extracellular matrix (ECM) [1].

The cellular population is integrated not only by adipocytes (the main cell type, by which receives its name) but also by preadipocytes, mesenchymal stem cells (MSCs), fibroblasts, endothelial and smooth muscle cells of blood vessels and any immune system cell, and adipose tissue macrophages (ATMs) with relevance [2, 3].

Its ECM, as any other, is composed of a wide type of collagens (fibrillar (I and III) and nonfibrillar (IV, VI, and VIII)), laminins, fibronectin, and proteoglycans; especially the external membrane contains a large complex of collagen IV and VIII as well as heparan sulfate proteoglycans and laminins [4]. AT ECM possesses the highest collagen VI concentration compared to any other body tissue [5, 6]. Altogether, the ECM and the non-adipocyte cellular population receive the name of stromal-vascular fraction (SVF) [7].

2.1.1 Classification

Histologically, AT is classified according to adipocyte microscopic characteristics as white (WAT), brown (BAT), and beige. White adipocytes are big oval cells with a single lipid droplet that fills the whole cytoplasm, displacing the nucleus and other organelles through periphery; its main function is the storage of energy in the form of triglycerides (TG) and lipolysis. Brown adipocytes are oval cells with multilocular lipid droplets uniformly distributed over the cytoplasm and have a high number of mitochondria, each one with several cristae expressing uncoupling protein 1 (UCP-1), characteristics that reflect an important thermogenic property. Beige adipocytes are cells with brown phenotype within WAT, that is why they are also called brite (brown-in-white) adipocytes; under basal conditions they express low quantity of UCP-1 but can overexpress it upon β-adrenergic simulation and thus acquire thermogenic function [8–10].

Moreover, adipose tissue has an important endocrine function, as it is capable to secrete own specific hormones called adipokines [11].

2.1.2 Fat depots

In humans WAT constitutes close to 5–10% of total human body weight and is located in two main compartments: intra-abdominal, named visceral AT (VAT), and subcutaneous AT (SCAT), also called hypodermis. VAT coats internal organs and protects them from mechanical friction and damage and can be divided into omental, mesenteric, retroperitoneal, gonadal and pericardial; SCAT is designated according to its superficial or deep situation regarding to the fascia superficialis as lamellar or areolar [12]. Moreover, abdominal and gluteofemoral regions are more relevant regarding of functional properties [13, 14].

It is remarkable to note that gender-related differences in distribution and quantity exist. While women have more SCAT (especially in gluteofemoral and peripheral regions), men have more VAT because SCAT has higher levels of estrogen and progesterone receptors, while VAT has more androgen receptors [15, 16].

In rodents, the main SCAT pads are anterior, from the neck to the axillae running through the interscapular area, and posterior, from the dorsolumbar to the gluteal region running through the inguinal region. Also, the striated muscle called *panniculus carnosus* clearly separates two layers of WAT depots: one directly underlying the reticular dermis and SCAT as such [17]; the former compartment is designated as dermal WAT (DWAT), composed primarily by intradermal adipocytes. These two terms were proposed as a redefinition of the nomenclature of skin-associated adipocytes, as it more accurately reflects their immediate developmental origin and anatomical location; humans, although not having a *panniculus carnosus*, possess functional and morphological distinctions between DWAT and SCAT [18, 19].

Differentiation, lipolytic and endocrine activity, and leucocyte population differ between VAT and SCAT, conferring them distinct metabolic properties and, in case of VAT, attribution of metabolic disturbances like dyslipidemia, glucose intolerance, and insulin resistance (IR) [20].

2.2 Immunometabolism

As an interdisciplinary field, immunometabolism emerged from discoveries of interdependent functions and mechanisms between the immune system and parenchymal cells of metabolic organs, which confer adaptive processes in homeostasis or disease at cellular, tissue, and systemic level [21, 22]. AT is the most studied in this field.

2.2.1 Immune response

Immune system has an important role on the control of AT homeostatic state, where its main functions are keeping an anti-inflammatory environment and remodeling of the extracellular matrix [8].

Under physiologic state, AT leucocyte population is integrated by eosinophils, mast cells, group 2 innate lymphoid cells (ILC2), invariant natural killer T cells (iNKT), regulatory T lymphocytes (Treg), and, of particular interest, adipose tissue macrophages (ATMs). It is proposed that these immune cells contribute to the maintenance of AT integrity through secretion of cytokines such as IL-4, IL-5, IL-13, and IL-10 (a Th2-type immune response) and that under hypercaloric state, macrophage accumulation may be a protective mechanism of the body to cope metabolic disturbances [23].

IL-33 produced by endothelial stromal cells has a key role in homeostatic maintenance and function of ECM. It is ligand of ST2 receptor, which is expressed in mast cells, Treg, eosinophils, ILC2s, and iNKT cells, practically the whole resident leucocyte population [24, 25].

In vitro and in vivo studies have demonstrated important effects of IL-33: production of IL-5 and IL-13 by Th2 lymphocytes and macrophages, eosinophil IL-4 production and survival, as well as ILC2s survival and expansion, the latter similar for Tregs [26]. iNKT cells express the transcriptional factor E4BP4; in adipose tissue produce anti-inflammatory cytokines, such as IL-2, IL-4, and IL-10; and participate in control of the homeostasis of Treg cells and macrophages in this tissue [27].

IL-25 promotes lipid metabolism and energy production, improves mitochondrial respiratory capacity, and alleviates lipid accumulation in the liver and AT via M2 macrophages and its interaction with adipocytes.

As we can observe, AT leucocytes produce the Th2-type cytokines, profile that favors the maintenance of ATMs in an anti-inflammatory M2 phenotype, known for the expression of arginase-1 (Arg-1, which inhibits iNOS activity) and production of IL-10 and IL-1Ra. ATMs also play an important lipid "buffering" activity, as they engulf free fatty acids (FFA) coming from adipocytes that have surpassed their lipid storage capacity and unchain lipolysis. Moreover, ATMs engulf death adipocytes that have reached a critical death size (CDS) [28] by a process named efferocytosis [29].

Thus, ATM is the fundamental leucocyte for correct AT functionality, as it engulfs apoptotic cell debris, and, FFA released whether by lipolysis or adipocyte death, promotes ECM reconstruction [30] and provides ECM components as scaffolds for its remodeling in the same way as under wound healing process; all these mechanisms promote adipogenesis and hyperplastic AT expansion. It is worth noting that these beneficial functions take place only under an anti-inflammatory M2 phenotype (**Figure 1**).

2.2.2 ECM remodeling

The ECM of any specialized connective tissue is essential not only for mechanic and structural sustain but also for providing a network that permits inter- and extracellular communication that enables proper growth and differentiation [1]. AT ECM is no exception, and its remodeling is regulated by resident leucocytes and own adipocytes.

WAT can undergo remodeling in response to changes in energy balance, like ECM degradation by members of the matrix metalloproteinase (MMP) family during adipocyte enlargement (hypertrophy) and allowing expansion by adipogenesis, under a positive energy balance [31, 32]; on the other hand, MMP activity counter-regulation is mediated by their tissue inhibitors (TIMPs). The balance between MMPs and TIMPs is critical for ECM integrity and function, and alterations in this proteolysis balance may contribute to many pathological states [33].

Secreted protein, acidic, and rich in cysteine complex (SPARC)/osteonectin and its C and N isoforms contribute to AT ECM remodeling; they modulate cell-ECM contact, cell-cell interaction, ECM deposition, and adipose stem cells (ASCs) migration and posterior incorporation into expanding neovasculature

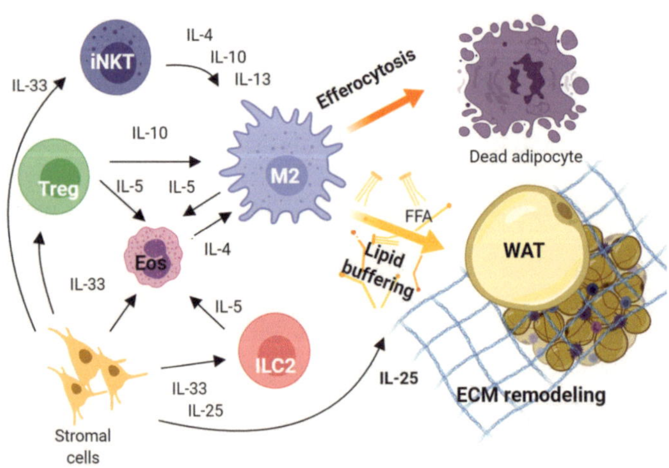

Figure 1.
Adipose tissue homeostatic immunometabolism.

accompanying WAT growth [34]. A study showed that serum concentrations of SPARC and MMP-2 after bariatric surgery decreased, SMAC correlated with HOMA-IR, and MMP-9 inversely correlated with serum adiponectin levels [35].

Regarding vasculature, AT ECM remodeling is influenced by a variety of angiogenic molecules, and it is triggered by transient hypoxia as a result of enlarged adipocytes under a positive energy balance. Hypoxia stimulates the production of angiogenic factors to compensate low perfusion rate; vascular endothelial growth factor (VEGF) is known as a master regulator of angiogenesis and plays crucial roles in the neovascular development of AT with obesity [36]. Hypoxia-inducible factor-1α (HIF-1α) binds to the proximal hypoxia response element in the *VEGF* gene promoter [37]; nevertheless, it also has a role in regulation of ECM remodeling, as overexpression of a constitutively active form of HIF-1α in adipose tissue forced the expression of pro-fibrotic genes, including *Col I* and *III*, *elastin*, *lysyl oxidase*, and *Timp1* [38].

This shows that detrimental ECM component deposition occurs under chronic hypoxic conditions. Transforming growth factor beta (TGFβ) and tumor necrosis factor-α (TNF-α) are released under acute hypoxia state and act as proangiogenic factors [39, 40], and the latter activates expression of preadipocyte genes in 3T3-L1 adipocytes [41]. This is in contrast to the belief that AT inflammation exerts a fundamentally negative impact on metabolism, postulating the concept "healthy inflammation" under overnutrition, requiring an acute local inflammation in order to prevent lipotoxicity and ectopic lipid accumulation; in this regard, a report showed the analysis of three animal models with constitutive or inducible expression of anti-inflammatory factors and revealed their inability to expand AT, leading to ectopic lipid deposition and deteriorated metabolic profile [42].

Platelet-derived growing factor B (PDGF-B), usually produced by endothelial cells, activates an intracellular signaling cascade binding to its receptor (PDGFRβ) and promotes pericyte detachment and migration around new-forming vessels for maturation, playing key roles in vascular development and wound healing in adults via angiogenic actions [43]. Surprisingly, Onogi Y. and colleagues found that M1 macrophages were a major type of cells expressing PDGF-B in obese adipose tissue and correlated with elevated pericyte detachment in a dose-dependent manner; in contrast, inducible knockout *pdgfrb* mice presented reduced M1 macrophages and CLS formation but increased M2 macrophages. Additionally, they were protected from body weight gain, accumulation of SCAT, VAT, and ectopic fat in muscle and liver and showed improved whole-body glucose metabolism under high-fat diet (HFD) condition. The expression of hypoxic and proinflammatory factors (*Hif1a, Emr1, Itgax, Mrc1, Tnfa, and Ccl2*) was significantly increased by HFD feeding mice, whereas the increasing effects were attenuated in HFD-fed *PDGFRB*-KO mice [44]. Also, increased adipogenic capacity of PDGFRβ+ precursors through *PPARG* overexpression in pericytes resulted in healthy VAT expansion in obesity and adiponectin-dependent improvements in glucose homeostasis, in contrast with knockout *PPARG* counterparts; moreover, the ability of the thiazolidinedione (TZD) class of antidiabetic drugs to promote healthy visceral WAT remodeling is dependent on mural cell *PPARG* [45].

An experimental in vivo study consisting of brown adipogenesis by β3-adrenergic receptor (ADRB3) activation caused crown-like structures (CLSs) formation: white adipocyte death recruited M2-polarized macrophages with high expression of osteopontin (OPN), which in turn attracted a subpopulation of PDGFRα+ CD44+ (OPN receptor) progenitors that underwent adipogenesis, in contrast with knockout OPN [46]. It is important to highlight that recruited M2 macrophages also showed upregulation of *Arg1* and *Il10* without significant changes in proinflammatory markers, indicating that ADRB3-mediated adipogenesis involves recruitment of macrophages that mediate non-inflammatory tissue repair [47]. Another study combining experiments in mouse models and human conditions reported that PDGFRα + $CD9^{high}$ cells originate pro-fibrotic cells, while their $CD9^{low}$ counterparts harbored pro-adipogenic potential; frequency of PDGFRα + $CD9^{high}$ in omental WAT (oWAT) correlated not only to oWAT fibrosis level but also to the severity of insulin resistance and T2D [48].

Adipokines can also help regulate angiogenesis, a sustained and progressive increase in leptin resulting from hypoxic conditions could induce VEGF and receptor (VEGFR2) expression, activate sirtuin 1 (SIRT1), and subsequent HIF-2α stabilization promoting its activity [49].

2.2.3 Glucose and lipid metabolism

A steady and continuous energy supply is necessary for all cells' survival; the production of the principal high-energy molecule, the adenosine triphosphate (ATP), is primarily obtained by the metabolism of such molecules as glucose and fatty acids. In the case of carbohydrates, these are the main source of energy in almost every living organism, from archaea to humans. It is not only the supply of these molecules, but also the intricate mechanism of regulation of pathways that control the consumption and storage of these biomolecules.

For example, after a meal, or what is called a post absorptive state, there is an increment of plasmatic glucose concentration which results in the secretion of hormones such as insulin by the pancreas; this contributes to the regulation of glucose metabolism as well, and the physiological response varies on every tissue, as can been seen in muscle and liver, where insulin favors glycolysis and glycogenesis. Nevertheless, this hormone not only alters the carbohydrates metabolism, but also promotes cholesterol synthesis and lipogenesis (or TG synthesis) in hepatic and adipose tissues [50].

In the case of glycolysis, it represents the central path for glucose metabolism and provides multiple intermediate products. On aerobic conditions, it starts in the cytoplasm of the cell, with glucose as a substrate, which is partially oxidized by 10 enzymatic reactions, obtaining two pyruvate molecules, reducing equivalents such as NADH (nicotinamide adenine dinucleotide in reduced form) and a net production of 2 ATPs for each glucose [51].

Afterward, the pyruvate molecules will be transformed into acetyl-CoA and transported into the mitochondria to continue their oxidation in the tricarboxylate cycle to produce two CO_2 molecules, three NADH and one FADH (flavin adenine dinucleotide in reduced form). The latter will transfer their electrons to the mitochondrial complexes of the electron respiratory chain; a series of redox transformation and the aid of molecular oxygen will finally converge in the synthesis of ATP by the ATP synthase complex.

Both ATP, NADH, and acetyl-CoA are metabolites that are shown to be thermodynamically favorable and are indicated as the protagonists in cellular energy metabolism [52].

After glycogen, the body stores energy in the form of TG in adipose tissue; nevertheless, diverse types of lipids are required for the maintenance of cellular functions, not only for energetic ones, but also structural (such as phospholipids) or for the formation of specialized products like steroid hormones. These are obtained from diet, absorbed and subsequently transported by lipoproteins such as the very high-density lipoprotein (VLDL), low-density lipoprotein (LDL) and high-density lipoprotein (HDL), all of these ensembled by the liver. FFAs are a major source of acetyl-CoA molecules by β-oxidation, these molecules continue their oxidation in the tricarboxylate cycle and the electron respiratory chain, providing a significant amount of energy at the cellular level.

Due to the importance of these biomolecules, there is a narrow regulation that includes transcription factors such as sterol regulatory element-binding proteins (SREBPs) and hormonal control for an adequate function [53].

Although these regulatory mechanisms are recognized, the possible regulatory activity that miRNAs may have in lipid and cholesterol homeostasis has recently been suggested, particularly for miR-122 and miR-33 [54].

3. Adipose tissue and disease

3.1 Insulin resistance

3.1.1 Obesity as a trigger

Obesity is a disease of multifactorial origin with a worldwide increasing prevalence; it entails an injurious health status for individuals, which represents a serious public health issue. This condition is associated to diverse diseases and has a complex treatment, being the reason why it must be assessed in a multidisciplinary context by healthcare professionals.

It is defined as an abnormal or excessive fat accumulation that can be detrimental for health [55]. It originates from the interrelation of inadequate food intake and/or overfeeding, sedentary lifestyle, and psychological, genetic, and ambiental factors. The excessive adiposity status hinders the disease reversion because of the difficulty to perform physical activity and the metabolic and satiety dysregulation [56].

Obesity develops a diversity of somatic complications such as respiratory, mechanic, cardiovascular, and metabolic, as well as psychological and social, which make its assessment, prognosis, and intervention even more complicated. Diagnosis is preceded by an anthropometric evaluation, which correlates adiposity with a total body weight of individuals [57].

Progressive AT expansion in the organism, given by a positive energy balance from excessive macronutrients and calorie intake, entails an elevated number of circulating FFA that triggers a deregulation in the organism, from changes in body structure to changes at local and systemic levels [58]. This excessive AT induces a chronic inflammatory state, also named lipoinflammation, causing hypoxia of adipocytes [59]. AT hypoxia and inflammation correlate with the risk of developing insulin resistance (IR), type 2 diabetes (T2D), and cardiovascular disease (CVD).

When the organism is under positive energy balance, energy excess accumulates in AT, giving place to SCAT hyperplasia until a physiologic allowed limit as energy reservoir is reached. When energy excess prevails, it is now stored at VAT; unfortunately this depot does not possess a great capacity as SCAT, resulting in adipocyte hypertrophy and subsequent android, central, or visceral adiposity [60, 61].

Central obesity is highly associated with T2D and CVD. AT is the pathogenic site where obesity-induced local IR originates before being systemic; its secretory genetic expression profile of endocrine and paracrine bioactive substances reflects a generalized inflammatory local state, the reason why adipocyte is referred to as key to the onset and development of obesity-induced inflammation and to macrophages as amplifiers of this process [62].

As aforementioned, AT initially plays a role in energy reservoir but also has a significant function in metabolism and immune system. Resident ATMs are key in IR onset, as they produce proinflammatory molecules which can explain more than

50% of secretion of TNF-α, by the action of insulin on adipocytes and on peripheric organs of the body [63].

Other implicated adipokines are resistin and IL-6, which stimulate hormone-sensitive lipase (HSL) activity resulting in triglycerides cleavage and subsequent glycerol and FFA release; these high circulating FFA levels are the cause and consequence of IR and T2D [64].

We can broadly elucidate that adipocytes and ATMs synthesize proinflammatory molecules and that weight increase at the expense of AT will contribute in turn to the perpetuation of chronic inflammation by increasing the levels of circulating cytokines. Required actions to help reverse the IR process should be focused on establishing a healthy diet accompanied by exercise; these will help to reduce the proinflammatory state, while downregulation of TNF-α and IL-6 expression of adipocytes occur. Meanwhile, exercise by its own will enhance mitochondrial FFA metabolism, avoiding their storage [65].

Other factors involved in IR and inflammation are implicated by diet and related to gut microbiota, which in turn demonstrates how an excessive saturated fat consumption can drive an important bacterial lipopolysaccharide (LPS) production, which impacts on systemic inflammation [58].

Initial steps that launch the inflammatory response are less well elucidated. On experimental studies with HFD-induced obesity murine models, HIF-1α levels are observed before the onset of a significant adiposity status; under this situation, adipocyte hypoxia and HIF-1α act as early triggers of inflammation and IR [59].

3.1.2 Inflammatory pathway

Adipose tissue complex and diverse functions have implications in the whole body, and cytokines are involved in his physiologic response. In obesity condition the major cytokines expressed by AT are leptin, resistin, TNFα, chemerin, MCP-1 and IL-6 [66, 67]. On the other hand, the adipose cells are both hyperplastic and hypertrophic, and in this state induce the inflammatory process. Dysregulation of adipose tissue promotes incorrect remodeling and subsequent inflammation, according to recruitment of macrophages and expression of chemotactic cytokines like MCP-1, TNFα and chemerin, to mention some of them. The phenotype involved is the M1 pro-inflammatory and evidence shows that this situation is not only local, but also systemic and this promotes further inflammation explaining how obesity can be the etiologic cause of other diseases [68, 69].

In addition, it is well known that this mechanism promotes insulin resistance, which is the previous phase before the development of T2D. However, the adipocyte is in a very close communication with the macrophage making the inflammatory process redundant and more complex. Nevertheless, in lean adipose tissue, it is typically the opposite, meaning that macrophages differentiate into a M2 anti-inflammatory phenotype, releasing IL-10, TGFβ, IL-4, and other regulatory cytokines [70]. Otherwise other mechanisms that can promote the anti-inflammatory pathway, like the consumption of Omega 3 fatty acids, exist [71].

Taking it all together, obesity results from genetic, epigenetic, physiological, behavioral, molecular and environmental factors that lead the proinflammatory phenotype [72, 73].

3.1.3 Molecular mechanism

It is described that adipose cells derive from a stem cell that can differentiate into adipocytes, chondrocytes, osteoblasts, and myocytes [74].

In a first phase, adipoblasts can be addressed to the adipogenic lineage and become preadipocytes. If the stimuli in the tissue continue, these cells maturate to become mature adipose cells with lipid storage capacity [75].

There are two main transcription factors that are involved in the differentiation of the adipocyte, CCAAT/enhancer-binding protein α (C/EBP-α), and peroxisome proliferator-activated receptor γ (PPAR-γ). PPAR-γ is the most described transcriptional factor, and its expression is regulated by the co-factor PGC1α and the production of adiponectin [76, 77].

Transcription factors that belong to the C/EBP family also have a crucial play in the differentiation, and there are reports that this factor can be activating more early than PPAR-γ (**Figure 2**) [78].

The dysfunction in the capacity of generating healthy adipose tissue has several metabolic consequences, like dyslipidemia, hypertension, and insulin resistance among others [79].

Many molecular mechanisms are involved since the adipocytes have different gene expression patterns, leading to the expression of different types of adipokines depending the phenotype induced in the tissue. Healthy expansion of adipocytes depends on the plasticity of the extracellular matrix, but in obesity there is a limiting in the oxygen diffusion, and it becomes hypoxic [80].

3.1.4 Role of adipokines and myokines

Skeletal muscle compounds 40% of total body weight in healthy individuals. The muscle is the major site for the insulin-stimulated glucose uptake and lipid metabolism, so it is an important part of metabolism maintenance [81].

Adipose tissue possesses more than 600 potentially secretory proteins, which means that more adipokines and myokines are still in line for discovery and characterization [82].

Additionally in adipokines there is a cross talk between these and myokines, which are synthetized by the muscle. Nevertheless, both tissues can express the same cytokines creating a regulation process with a strong communication. The most characterized cytokines are chemerin, TNFa, MCP-1 and IL-6. It is demonstrated that WAT deposits exist in skeletal muscle and facilitate communication, also, these tissues usually are in close anatomical proximity.

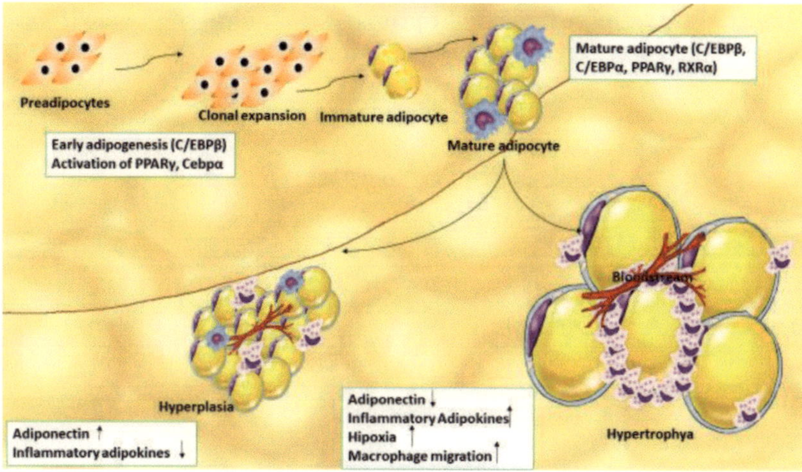

Figure 2.
Adipose tissue differentiation and hyperplasia and hypertrophy consequences.

The knowledge of the most important characterized myokines is as follows:

IL-6: this increases in favor of the exercises, but it is recognized that it has a controversial role in the inflammatory or anti-inflammatory pathway.

Il-15: it mediates a beneficial effect on physical activity.

Irisin: it stimulates the development of brown adipose tissue activating MPK and ERK molecular ways, and it is regulated by the age and gender. This molecule has also a controversial role, because it has been reported to increase obesity.

Myonectin: it has a homology worth the sequence of adiponectin and promotes fatty acid uptaking in mice [82, 84–86].

Principally, the major role of the adipomyokines is contributing to metabolism, angiogenesis, blood vessel regulation, adipogenesis, myogenesis, and immune response [82]. On the other hand, it is important to remark the impact that macrophages have in metabolism, since they induce a response in both tissues. For example, when circulating monocytes respond to chemoattractant molecules, they migrate into adipose and muscle tissue, and then develop a phenotype depending on environmental necessities (**Table 1**) [94].

Finally, there is another terminology newly adopted by the scientist called organokines, because it has been suggested that all proteins secreted in various tissues or organs (liver, adipose tissue, muscle, and bone) have an intimate relationship in the context of the communication and regulation for the maintaining of homeostasis and that they are involved in a network of paracrine and endocrine cross talk [84].

3.1.5 Emerging role of microRNAs in obesity

In the context of complex diseases, obesity is the prototype of immunometabolic disease; it is considered a major factor that triggers metabolic risk and the development of secondary chronic illness[2], insulin resistance (IR), and metabolic syndrome (MS). The susceptibility of a subject to develop obesity will depend on different factors such as the repertoire of individual variations in an ensemble of relevant genes, their history of exposure to environmental risk factors, and the interaction between the lifestyle and metabolism, which is also modulated by the gene regulators [95–97].

Meanwhile, obesity presents many subclinical manifestations, characterized by alterations in lipids and carbohydrate metabolism at different levels; most of these changes is due to a low-grade systemic chronic inflammation [98, 99] that favors the development of IR. Adipose tissue is the primary anatomical site where IR disease takes place; in early stage this tissue became inflamed.

IL-6	[87]
IL-8	[88]
MCP-1	[89]
Irisin	[82]
PAI-1	[90]
PEDF	[91]
FGF21	[92]
Fstl 1	[93]

Table 1.
Best characterized adipomyokines.

Novel findings on the immune-regulatory processes and metabolic mechanisms may open new avenues in the treatment of the common complex diseases as well as inflammatory component; research on basic and clinical advances in immunometabolism has evolved rapidly during the past years, and the beginning of new tools for the detection and characterization of regulation of inflammation in metabolic diseases with comorbidity may play an imperative role; nevertheless, the precise mechanisms mediating this relationship remains poorly understood.

Interplay in the regulation of inflammation and metabolic risk factors are a complex cluster. The inflammatory condition associated with adipose tissue represents a triggering factor in the etiology of the obesity pathological mechanisms and mainly contributes to the related disease outcomes.

In the early stages of obesity, in white adipose tissue, primed immune cells are recruited as adiposity increases, and these cells became resident cells (mainly macrophages) and secrete proinflammatory adipokines that promote further recruitment of circulating monocytes [100–103]. Later, they polarize toward M1 macrophages, favoring a subclinical chronic inflammatory state [102, 104–106] secondary to irregular increase and distribution of fat depots [107]. In IR, the expression of genes implicated in glucose and lipid absorption and metabolism in liver and adipose tissue is dysregulated, at the same time, insulin signaling pathway in peripheral tissues is also disturbed [108]; this IR scenario precedes the development of T2D and other related diseases.

The identification of diverse molecular mechanisms related to energy metabolism has allowed the definition of strategies for searching genes implied in obesity and IR.

In the decade that precedes us, experimental reports show the existence of small noncoding RNAs, which are identified as microRNAs, (miRs) with the function of regulating cellular processes through modulating the expression of genes that code for functional proteins.

The insulin signaling pathways may be regulated by microRNAs (miRNA) that modulate the stability and translation of messenger RNAs (mRNA) by a particular mechanism of binding seeding sequences located in target genes, resulting in protein decay [109, 110].

Once synthesized, some miRNA can be released into circulation via exosomes, vesicular bodies, lipoproteins, simple extrusion, or apoptotic bodies. Most researches in the field have assessed the presence of circulating miRNA in many body fluids, being related to their impaired expression in tissues under physiological and pathological conditions. Several studies have shown a correlation of particular circulating miRNA with the development of different pathologies, positioning them as valuable biomarkers in silent diseases such as obesity, IR, and MS [111, 112].

Although rapid progress is being made in research on miRs, there is little availability of experimental tools with scientific value and mechanisms that lead from the discoveries of miRs to the therapeutic application in diseases. Therefore, the current demand is to explore the expression and biological function of miRs in the development of diseases in vivo.

The main considerations that are known are that the process of its biogenesis is governed by regulatory checkpoints, based on the fact that the sequence of the primary transcript does not correspond linearly to mature miR. The abundance or scarcity of a miR indicates its level of regulation.

Under physiological conditions, it has been shown that miRs modulate gene expression; however pathological stress increases or decreases its function. Therefore, its function will be defined by the effect on the expression of the genes to which it is directed. Predictions indicate that 60% of target mRNA genes have similar binding sequences in the 3′UTR region for single or multiple miRs. These miRs exert their silencing function through two different mechanisms: translation inhibition (initiation or elongation) and target mRNA degradation. In the target genes for miRs, it is observed that 3′UTR regions have binding sites for multiple miRs; this suggests cooperation and redundancy of the effect on gene expression between the different miRs.

Currently, there are 1917 human miRNAs listed in the miRNA database miRBase (http://www.mirbase.org), representing 1% of all genes in the human genome. These miRNAs are predicted to target aprox. 30% of the human gene pool.

From the extraction of plasma and blood serum miRs from human and mammalian animal samples, they have been proposed as diagnostic biomarkers in the diseases. The attributes that stand out are that the miRs extracted from the serum have stability, and the results in the quantification are reproducible and consistent among individuals of the same species.

The logical sequence in the integral investigation of miRs is firstly to identify the presence in a given sample. The experimental tools used to measure the expression profile of miRs have been by microarray analysis or deep sequencing, while the determination of the level of expression of individual miRs has been performed by RT-PCR, in situ hybridization or northern blot.

However, the investigations carried out can be categorized from two conceptual points, the determination of the level of expression in which the most used methodological tool is real-time PCR analysis and global expression assays. The former stand out for their specificity while confirming the latter, while the latter provide a broad view of the presence and regulation of miRs.

Properly identifying the functionality and level of expression of a specific miR is limited due to the high degree of sequence homology between some miRs and the size of the molecule; the parallel application of different molecular tools strengthens the identification or quantification process of the level of expression. However, an unfavorable factor is the combined regulation of multiple genes or small changes in gene regulation that are lost in biological noise.

Enhancing the work of performing research surrounding these novel gene regulators will advance our understanding of miRNAs and their specific functions and will augment the opportunities to safely follow them as therapeutic targets [113].

3.2 IR in muscle and liver

Conventionally, insulin acts directly on the WAT under the cascade of the IRS1 axis, PI3K, and AKT, for glucose absorption, with a possible positive feedback of the phosphorylation of Ser^{388} from IRS2, by cyclin-dependent kinase 4 (CDK4) [114], culminating with lipolysis regulation. However, as described in previous sections of the chapter, inflammatory processes and alternative activation of macrophages favor the pathogenic adiposity in which the action of insulin is not carried out correctly and therefore does not slow the lipolysis process.

Although the mechanism of signaling pathways that links pathogenic adiposity to insulin resistance in skeletal muscle and liver has not been well defined due to the difficulty of modeling in vitro systems that allow cell coordination as in a complex organism, the process of understanding molecular bases has lagged behind the direct action of insulin in an organ or cell. The best way to associate it is the chronic surplus of energy that favors the accumulation of ectopic lipids in the liver and skeletal muscle that trigger the activation of pathways that impair insulin signaling, causing the decrease in glucose absorption in muscle cells and of glycogenesis in liver [115].

3.2.1 Liver

In a physiological stage with food withdrawal, the main source of glucose in the bloodstream is the liver. On the other hand, after absorption of nutrients by the intestine, the production of hepatic glucose should be interrupted in coordination with hyperinsulinemia.

The most assertive explanations of how insulin acts to promote glucose homeostasis by inhibiting both glycogenolysis and hepatic gluconeogenesis have focused on the canonical pathway of insulin interacting directly in the liver by activating the insulin receptor (InsR) and the substrate of insulin receptor (IRS) and the phosphoinositol 3-kinase signaling cascade (PI3K/Akt/mTOR pathway) by inhibiting transcription of the forkhead box class O-1FOXO1 factor and thus gene transcription and activation of gluconeogenic enzymes such as phosphoenolpyruvate carboxykinase (PCK1) and glucose 6 phosphatase (G6PC) [116, 117].

However, it has been observed that suppression of hepatic glucose production is not totally dependent on the Akt activation pathway, for which remote insulin actions that interact indirectly with the physiological process of hepatic glucose have been studied. On one hand, the reduction of PCK1 and glucose 6-phosphatase (G6Pase) through cerebral insulin action activates the ATP-sensitive potassium channels (K_{ATP}) of hypothalamus and stimulate the vagal transmission and STAT3 activation [118, 119], blocking the *de novo* glucose formation by the liver and therefore regulating serum hyperglycemia.

On the other hand, insulin action in WAT suppresses lipolysis and reduces the fatty acids flow into the liver, therefore, reduction of both acetyl-CoA concentration and pyruvate-to-glucose conversion occur, corresponding with the cessation of glycerol supply, observing a decrease in pyruvate carboxylase (PC) enzyme activity [120].

However, when WAT is in an inflammatory process and insulin resistance, it constantly increases the supply of gluconeogenic substrates, such as non-esterified fatty acids (NEFAS), and glycerol favors hepatic glucose production [121]. In stages with normal insulin levels, fatty acids in the bloodstream compete with glucose to internalize cells independent of hyperglycemia; however when insulin concentration or activity is deficient, fatty acids contribute directly to the production of glucose [122]. The ectopic accumulation of fatty acids in liver increases the content of acetyl-CoA allosterically activating PC and increasing gluconeogenesis; this increase in glucose and the presence of pro-inflammatory cytokines lead to inadequate insulin signaling in liver and subsequently, IR [123].

According to current knowledge of the importance of indirect insulin pathways in the liver to maintain the homeostatic glucose process, research groups will follow some therapeutic targets associated with the signaling pathways of G-protein-coupled receptors (GPCRs) [124] as well as inhibitors of the enzyme acetyl-CoA carboxylase [125, 126] for the treatment of metabolic diseases. Similarly there is evidence that proves that the diet with low calorie concentrations can reverse hyperglycemia [127].

3.2.2 Muscle

The skeletal muscle is responsible for 70% of the elimination of total body glucose, associated with its capacity and energy need. Therefore, insulin sensitivity of skeletal muscle is critically important in maintaining homeostasis of blood glucose [128].

Many studies propose molecules related to the deterioration in insulin signaling; however, they agree that these molecules accumulate when the energy supply exceeds the demand in the body. Therefore, it suggests that the IR in the muscle not only has intrinsic problems as a reference. One of the main mechanisms proposed to elucidate the pathogenic process of IR in skeletal muscle is mitochondrial compromise due to the bioenergetic imbalance present mainly in pathological adiposity. However, the molecular pathways to describe this event are not entirely elucidated.

In the physiological process of insulin/IR interaction in skeletal muscle, you can activate two signaling pathways with the phosphorylation of IRS1 and, on the one hand, the PI3K/AKT pathway that induces glycogen synthesis and glucose uptake by recruiting the transporter protein of glucose (GLUT-4) to the plasma membrane, while the activation of the MAPK pathway favors the growth and differentiation of skeletal muscle [129].

The presence of pathological adiposity provides high concentrations of fatty acids and cytokines that activate signaling pathways linked to obesity that converge with insulin signaling. As plasma FFA increase, they accumulate in muscle. Intramuscular diacylglycerol (DAG) and ceramides levels rise, compounds that might act as second messengers in alternative signaling pathways that interfere with IRS-1 adequate phosphorylation [108, 130].

The presence of TAG and DG in muscle activates Ser^{307} phosphorylation in IRS-1, resulting in the activation of PKC-θ. These changes in turn result in a decrease in the tyrosine phosphorylation of IRS-1 and a lower activation of the PI3K associated with IRS-1, resulting in a decrease in insulin-stimulated glucose transport activity. Intramolecular lipids (IMCL) have been observed to be elevated when lipid oxidation is poor and lipid supply to the muscle is exceeded [120, 131, 132].

The bioenergetic imbalance favors mitochondrial beta oxidation, although incompletely which can increase the concentration of reactive oxygen species (ROS) mainly H_2O_2, this reactive species is responsible for the inhibition of PP2A causing the activation of JNK and ERK, and these inhibit serine phosphorylation in IRS1. When the energy demand is exceeded, skeletal muscle mitochondria stimulate lipid biosynthesis that redundantly increases the concentration of ROS and myocellular lipids [133–135].

Although the process by which ROS and fatty acids trigger insulin resistance is not yet elucidated, it can be deduced that energy imbalance is the fundamental key.

4. A new terminology: pathologic adiposity

Total adipose mass, fat depot location, and particular AT type function are the predominant factors that explain high metabolic risk in individuals with obesity, since number, distribution, and leucocyte population differ between SCAT and VAT from lean and obese individuals; VAT has higher a macrophage number, and adipocyte size is smaller and has less lipid storage capacity. These differences suggest VAT can undergo subclinical inflammation and metabolic disease [136]; actually, central obesity associates with higher CVD, metabolic disorders, and early death, in contrast with gynecoid obesity at the expense of SCAT accumulation in the gluteofemoral region [13].

With the aforementioned, we can state that not every obese individual is affected by the common metabolic abnormalities associated with obesity. Approximately 10–25% of obese and a smaller fraction of morbidly obese persons are "metabolically healthy" (metabolically healthy obese, MHO), as they are insulin sensitive and normotensive and possess a favorable lipid profile; furthermore, they present less VAT and hepatic lipids and possess normal glucose metabolism. On the other hand, a subgroup of normal weight individuals suffers obesity characteristic metabolic abnormalities, whereby they are denominated as "metabolically healthy

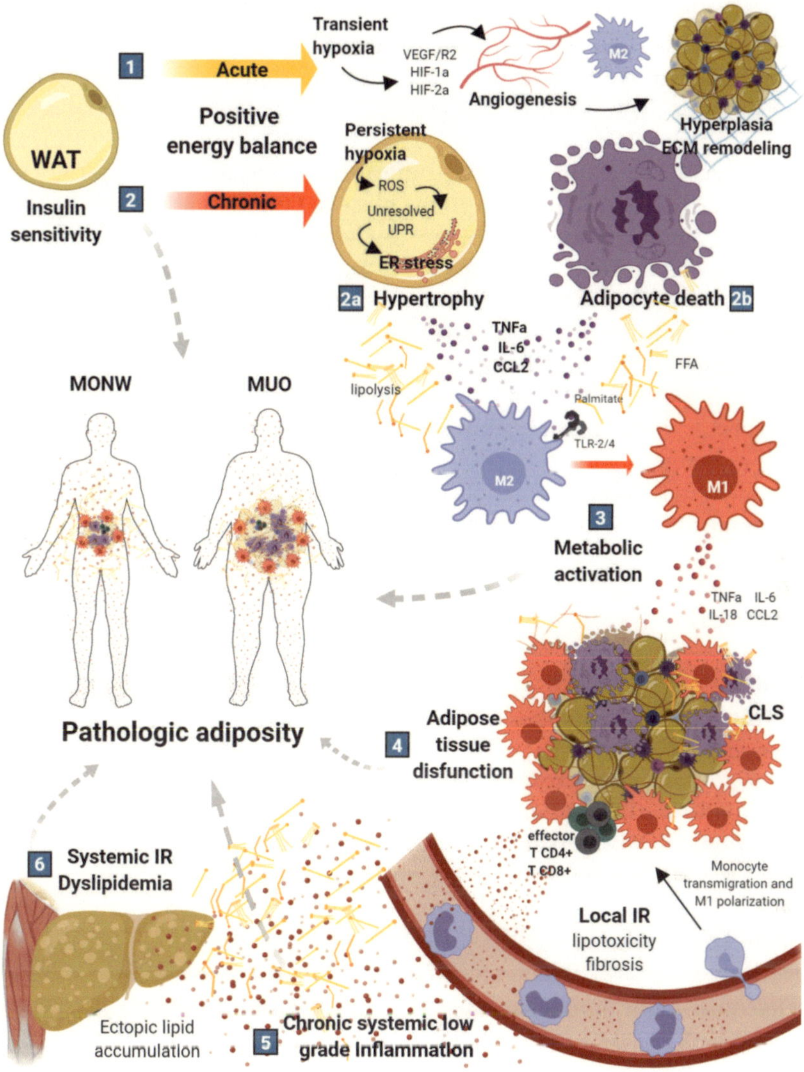

Figure 3.
A series of unfortunate events that leads to a pathologic adiposity status.

but with normal weight" (MONW). It is suggested that MHO individuals own a less detrimental metabolic profile and better prognosis compared to normal weight individuals with metabolic syndrome [137–139].

As stated before in this chapter, under acute caloric excess, enlarged adipocytes suffer hypoperfusion and mechanic stress owing to its surrounding ECM, which causes transient hypoxia and triggers angiogenesis and release of stress signals so that AT could undergo healthy remodeling and maintenance [140].

Nonetheless, obesity is a chronic caloric excess state, which means adipocyte enlargement surpasses angiogenesis, whereby hypoxia and stress signals perpetuate and cause fibrosis and cell death with eventual necrosis; this scenario causes local lipotoxicity, as ATM lipid buffering function is surpassed by the increased FFAs levels caused by overfeeding or adipocyte lipolysis and death [141, 142]. Thus, ATMs undergo metabolic activation, as lipids like palmitate are TLR-2/4 ligands, therefore initiating a proinflammatory response and polarization towards a M1 phenotype, losing all pro-homeostatic functions that we have previously discussed [143–145].

Furthermore, the other resident leucocytes will change in number and function as ATMs did, towards a Th1-type immune response.

The activation of NF-kB pathway with cytokine/chemokine release and the contribution of harmful metabolites (i.e., ceramide and sphingosine 1-phosphate, S1P) interfere with proper insulin signaling, therefore establishing a local AT IR [146–148].

After the AT IR is established, non-suppressive lipolysis now perpetuates and triggers high circulating FFA levels giving place to peripheral/systemic lipotoxicity: ectopic fat accumulation in liver and muscle; additionally, the proinflammatory cytokine, adipokine, and chemokine profile will circulate through the bloodstream, establishing metainflammation. Eventually, the high ectopic lipid concentration in this tissues will unleash similar detrimental effects that took place at AT, establishing now peripheral/systemic IR and dyslipidemia [132, 149].

The ensemble of this AT dysfunction and its harmful metabolic clinical repercussions is what we call pathologic adiposity: the adiposity status that determinates metabolic systemic dysfunction (IR and dyslipidemia), whether in an obese or normal weight individual, "metabolically unhealthy obese" (MUO), or "metabolically obese normal weight" (MONW) person, respectively (**Figure 3**).

5. Conclusions

Metainflammation can be defined as the systemic metabolic inflammation derived from obese adipose tissue in which innate and adaptive immune system cells have changed in number and function, from a lean and homeostatic to a proinflammatory state, and whose cytokine and adipokine proinflammatory profiles cause metabolic syndrome. Some authors consider metainflammation as the result of dysfunctional adipose tissue that consists of unhealthy expansion (hypertrophy) and angiogenesis, hypoxia, and detrimental ECM remodeling, which in turn limit adipocyte lipid storage capacity; altogether, these deleterious scenarios cause lipolysis and ectopic fat accumulation in the liver and muscle.

The knowledge developed in recent years in relation to the homeostatic interaction between immune system and the energetic metabolism along with the role of miRs allows that in a state in imbalance such as obesity, new biomarkers that show clinical information about the state are sought health of individuals and the early detection of the risk of developing metabolic complications is derived from the state of pathological adiposity.

Conflict of interest

The authors declare no conflict of interest.

Acronyms and abbreviations

ADRB3	β3-adrenergic receptor
AKT	protein kinase B
ASCs	adipose stem cells
AT	adipose tissue
ATMs	adipose tissue macrophages
ATP	adenosine triphosphate
BAT	brown adipose tissue
C/EBP-α	CCAAT/enhancer-binding protein α

CDK4	cyclin-dependent kinase 4
CDS	critical death size
CVD	cardiovascular disease
DWAT	dermal WAT
ECM	extracellular matrix
ERK	extracellular signal-regulated kinase-1
FADH	flavin adenine dinucleotide in reduced form
FFA	free fatty acids
FGF21	fibroblast growth factor 21
FOXO1	forkhead box class O-1
Fstl 1	follistatin-related protein 1
G6PaseC	glucose 6 phosphatase
GLUT	transporter protein of glucose
HDL	high-density lipoproteins
HFD	high-fat diet
HIF-1α	hypoxia-inducible factor-1α
HSL	hormone sensitive lipase
IL	interleukin
ILC2	group 2 innate lymphoid cells
IMCL	intramolecular lipids
iNKT	invariant natural killer T cells
IR	insulin resistance
IRS1	substrate of insulin receptor 1
IRS2	substrate of insulin receptor 2
K_{ATP}	ATP-sensitive potassium channels
LDL	low-density lipoprotein
LPS	lipopolysaccharide
MCP-1	monocyte chemoattractant protein-1
miRs	microRNAs
MPK	mitogen-activated protein kinase
mRNA	messenger RNAs
MS	metabolic syndrome
MSCs	mesenchymal stem cells
NADH	nicotinamide adenine dinucleotide in reduced form
NEFAS	non-esterified fatty acids
OPN	osteopontin
PAI-1	plasminogen activator inhibitor-1
PCK1	phosphoenolpyruvate carboxy kinase
PC	pyruvate carboxylase
PDGF	platelet-derived growth factor
PDGFR	platelet-derived growth factor receptor
PEDF	pigment epithelium-derived factor
PI3K	phosphoinositide 3-kinases
PPAR-γ	peroxisome proliferator-activated receptor γ
RT-PCR	real-time polymerase chain reaction
SCAT	subcutaneous adipose tissue
SIRT 1	sirtuin 1
SPARC	secreted protein, acidic, and rich in cysteine complex
SREBPs	sterol regulatory element-binding proteins
STAT3	signal transducer and activator of transcription 3
SVF	stromal-vascular fraction
S1P	sphingosine-1-phosphate
TZD	thiazolidinediones

TIMP	tissue inhibitor of matrix metalloproteinases
T2D	type 2 diabetes
TG	triglycerides
TGFβ	transforming growth factor beta
TNFα	tumor necrosis factor alpha
Treg	regulatory T lymphocytes
UCP-1	uncoupling protein 1
VAT	visceral adipose tissue
VLDL	very-low-density lipoprotein
WAT	white adipose tissue

Author details

Fernanda-Isadora Corona-Meraz[1,2], Jesus-Aureliano Robles-De Anda[1,3], Perla-Monserrat Madrigal-Ruiz[1], Gustavo-Ignacio Díaz-Rubio[3], Jorge Castro-Albarrán[1,4] and Rosa-Elena Navarro-Hernández[1*]

1 UDG-CA-701, Research Group on Immunometabolism and Complex Diseases, Department of Molecular Biology and Genomics, Health Sciences School, University of Guadalajara, Guadalajara, Jalisco, Mexico

2 Department of Biomedical Sciences, Health Sciences Division, CUTonalá, University of Guadalajara, Tonalá, Jalisco, Mexico

3 Doctoral Program in Molecular Sciences in Medicine, Department of Molecular Biology and Genomics, Health Sciences School, University of Guadalajara, Guadalajara, Jalisco, Mexico

4 Department of Health Sciences and Human Ecology, Regional Development Division, CUCSur, University of Guadalajara, Autlán de Navarro, Jalisco, Mexico

*Address all correspondence to: rosa_elena_n@hotmail.com

References

[1] Ross M, Wojciech P. Connective tissue. In: Histology: A Text and Atlas with Correlated Cell and Molecular Biology. Philadelphia: Wolters Kluwer/Lippincott Williams & Wilkins Health; 2015. p. 992

[2] Haylett WL, Ferris WF. Adipocyte-progenitor cell communication that influences adipogenesis. Cellular and Molecular Life Sciences. 2019. Available from: https://doi.org/10.1007/s00018-019-03256-5

[3] Russo L, Lumeng CN. Properties and functions of adipose tissue macrophages in obesity. Immunology. 2018;**155**(4):407-417

[4] Martinez-Santibanez G, Lumeng CN. Macrophages and the regulation of adipose tissue remodeling. Annual Review of Nutrition. 2014;**34**:57-76

[5] Khan T et al. Metabolic dysregulation and adipose tissue fibrosis: Role of collagen VI. Molecular and Cellular Biology. 2009;**29**(6):1575-1591

[6] Pasarica M et al. Adipose tissue collagen VI in obesity. The Journal of Clinical Endocrinology and Metabolism. 2009;**94**(12):5155-5162

[7] Orr JS, Kennedy AJ, Hasty AH. Isolation of adipose tissue immune cells. Journal of Visualized Experiments. 2013;**75**:e50707

[8] Rodriguez A et al. Revisiting the adipocyte: A model for integration of cytokine signaling in the regulation of energy metabolism. American Journal of Physiology. Endocrinology and Metabolism. 2015;**309**(8):E691-E714

[9] Ross M, Wojciech P. Adipose tissue. In: Histology: A Text and Atlas with Correlated Cell and Molecular Biology. Philadelphia: Wolters Kluwer/Lippincott Williams & Wilkins Health; 2015. p. 992

[10] Zwick RK et al. Anatomical, physiological, and functional diversity of adipose tissue. Cell Metabolism. 2018;**27**(1):68-83

[11] Fasshauer M, Bluher M. Adipokines in health and disease. Trends in Pharmacological Sciences. 2015;**36**(7):461-470

[12] Stenkula KG, Erlanson-Albertsson C. Adipose cell size: Importance in health and disease. American Journal of Physiology. Regulatory, Integrative and Comparative Physiology. 2018;**315**(2):R284-r295

[13] Goossens GH. The metabolic phenotype in obesity: Fat mass, body fat distribution, and adipose tissue function. Obesity Facts. 2017;**10**(3):207-215

[14] Fitzgerald SJ et al. A new approach to study the sex differences in adipose tissue. Journal of Biomedical Science. 2018;**25**(1):89

[15] Chang E, Varghese M, Singer K. Gender and sex differences in adipose tissue. Current Diabetes Reports. 2018;**18**(9):69

[16] Blouin K et al. Effects of androgens on adipocyte differentiation and adipose tissue explant metabolism in men and women. Clinical Endocrinology. 2010;**72**(2):176-188

[17] Totowa AO. In: Mazzone T, Fantuzzi G, editors. Nutrition and Health: Adipose Tissue and Adipokines in Health and Disease. Chicago, Il, USA: Springer; 2007. pp. 3-19

[18] Schmidt B, Horsley V. Unravelling hair follicle-adipocyte communication. Experimental Dermatology. 2012;**21**(11):827-830

[19] Driskell RR et al. Defining dermal adipose tissue. Experimental Dermatology. 2014;**23**(9):629-631

[20] Wajchenberg BL. Subcutaneous and visceral adipose tissue: Their relation to the metabolic syndrome. Endocrine Reviews. 2000;**21**(6):697-738

[21] Kohlgruber AC, LaMarche NM, Lynch L. Adipose tissue at the nexus of systemic and cellular immunometabolism. Seminars in Immunology. 2016;**28**(5):431-440

[22] Man K, Kutyavin VI, Chawla A. Tissue immunometabolism: Development, physiology, and pathobiology. Cell Metabolism. 2017;**25**(1):11-26

[23] Dalmas E. Role of innate immune cells in metabolism: From physiology to type 2 diabetes. Seminars in Immunopathology. 2019;**41**(4):531-545

[24] Ferrante AW Jr. The immune cells in adipose tissue. Diabetes, Obesity & Metabolism. 2013;**15**(Suppl 3):34-38

[25] Ghazarian M et al. Immunopathology of adipose tissue during metabolic syndrome. Turk Patoloji Dergisi. 2015;**31**(Suppl 1): 172-180

[26] de Oliveira MFA, Talvani A, Rocha-Vieira E. IL-33 in obesity: Where do we go from here? Inflammation Research. 2019;**68**(3):185-194

[27] Satoh M, Iwabuchi K. Communication between natural killer T cells and adipocytes in obesity. Adipocytes. 2016;**5**(4):389-393

[28] Cinti S. Reversible physiological transdifferentiation in the adipose organ. The Proceedings of the Nutrition Society. 2009;**68**(4):340-349

[29] Cash JG et al. Apolipoprotein E4 impairs macrophage efferocytosis and potentiates apoptosis by accelerating endoplasmic reticulum stress. The Journal of Biological Chemistry. 2012;**287**(33):27876-27884

[30] Cai J et al. Macrophage infiltration regulates the adipose ECM reconstruction and the fibrosis process after fat grafting. Biochemical and Biophysical Research Communications. 2017;**490**(2):560-566

[31] Bauters D et al. Gelatinase A (MMP-2) promotes murine adipogenesis. Biochimica et Biophysica Acta. 2015;**1850**(7):1449-1456

[32] Bouloumie A et al. Adipocyte produces matrix metalloproteinases 2 and 9: Involvement in adipose differentiation. Diabetes. 2001;**50**(9):2080-2086

[33] Chavey C et al. Matrix metalloproteinases are differentially expressed in adipose tissue during obesity and modulate adipocyte differentiation. The Journal of Biological Chemistry. 2003;**278**(14):11888-11896

[34] Tseng C, Kolonin MG. Proteolytic isoforms of SPARC induce adipose stromal cell mobilization in obesity. Stem Cells. 2016;**34**(1):174-190

[35] Lee YJ et al. Serum SPARC and matrix metalloproteinase-2 and metalloproteinase-9 concentrations after bariatric surgery in obese adults. Obesity Surgery. 2014;**24**(4):604-610

[36] Sung HK et al. Adipose vascular endothelial growth factor regulates metabolic homeostasis through angiogenesis. Cell Metabolism. 2013;**17**(1):61-72

[37] He Q et al. Regulation of HIF-1{alpha} activity in adipose tissue by obesity-associated factors: Adipogenesis, insulin, and hypoxia. American Journal of Physiology. Endocrinology and Metabolism. 2011;**300**(5):E877-E885

[38] Halberg N et al. Hypoxia-inducible factor 1alpha induces fibrosis and insulin resistance in white adipose

tissue. Molecular and Cellular Biology. 2009;**29**(16):4467-4483

[39] Zubkova ES et al. Regulation of adipose tissue stem cells angiogenic potential by tumor necrosis factor-alpha. Journal of Cellular Biochemistry. 2016;**117**(1):180-196

[40] Li J et al. Gene expression profile of rat adipose tissue at the onset of high-fat-diet obesity. American Journal of Physiology. Endocrinology and Metabolism. 2002;**282**(6):E1334-E1341

[41] Ruan H et al. Tumor necrosis factor-alpha suppresses adipocyte-specific genes and activates expression of preadipocyte genes in 3T3-L1 adipocytes: Nuclear factor-kappaB activation by TNF-alpha is obligatory. Diabetes. 2002;**51**(5):1319-1336

[42] Wernstedt Asterholm I et al. Adipocyte inflammation is essential for healthy adipose tissue expansion and remodeling. Cell Metabolism. 2014;**20**(1):103-118

[43] Andrae J, Gallini R, Betsholtz C. Role of platelet-derived growth factors in physiology and medicine. Genes & Development. 2008;**22**(10):1276-1312

[44] Onogi Y et al. PDGFRbeta regulates adipose tissue expansion and glucose metabolism via vascular remodeling in diet-induced obesity. Diabetes. 2017;**66**(4):1008-1021

[45] Shao M et al. De novo adipocyte differentiation from Pdgfrbeta(+) preadipocytes protects against pathologic visceral adipose expansion in obesity. Nature Communications. 2018;**9**(1):890

[46] Lee YH, Petkova AP, Granneman JG. Identification of an adipogenic niche for adipose tissue remodeling and restoration. Cell Metabolism. 2013;**18**(3):355-367

[47] Murray PJ, Wynn TA. Protective and pathogenic functions of macrophage subsets. Nature Reviews. Immunology. 2011;**11**(11):723-737

[48] Marcelin G et al. A PDGFRalpha-mediated switch toward CD9(high) adipocyte progenitors controls obesity-induced adipose tissue fibrosis. Cell Metabolism. 2017;**25**(3):673-685

[49] Delle Monache S et al. Adipose-derived stem cells sustain prolonged angiogenesis through leptin secretion. Growth Factors. 2016;**34**(3-4):87-96

[50] Chao HW et al. Homeostasis of glucose and lipid in non-alcoholic fatty liver disease. International Journal of Molecular Sciences. 2019;**20**(2):1-18. Available from: http://dx.doi.org/10.3390/ijms20020298

[51] Lenzen S. A fresh view of glycolysis and glucokinase regulation: History and current status. The Journal of Biological Chemistry. 2014;**289**(18):12189-12194

[52] Walsh CT, Tu BP, Tang Y. Eight kinetically stable but thermodynamically activated molecules that power cell metabolism. Chemical Reviews. 2018;**118**(4):1460-1494

[53] Raghow R et al. SREBPs: The crossroads of physiological and pathological lipid homeostasis. Trends in Endocrinology and Metabolism. 2008;**19**(2):65-73

[54] Rottiers V, Naar AM. MicroRNAs in metabolism and metabolic disorders. Nature Reviews. Molecular Cell Biology. 2012;**13**(4):239-250

[55] Obesity: Preventing and managing the global epidemic. Report of a WHO consultation. World Health Organization Technical Report Series. 2000;**894**:i-xii, 1-253

[56] Sangros FJ et al. Association of general and abdominal obesity with

hypertension, dyslipidemia and prediabetes in the PREDAPS study. Revista Española de Cardiología. 2018;**71**(3):170-177

[57] Faucher P et al. Bariatric surgery in obese patients with type 1 diabetes: Effects on weight loss and metabolic control. Obesity Surgery. 2016;**26**(10):2370-2378

[58] Barazzoni R et al. Insulin resistance in obesity: An overview of fundamental alterations. Eating and Weight Disorders. 2018;**23**(2):149-157

[59] Lee YS et al. Increased adipocyte O_2 consumption triggers HIF-1alpha, causing inflammation and insulin resistance in obesity. Cell. 2014;**157**(6):1339-1352

[60] Bosch TA et al. Identification of sex-specific thresholds for accumulation of visceral adipose tissue in adults. Obesity (Silver Spring). 2015;**23**(2):375-382

[61] Rachel Marie Watson PRS, Talley AE, Stults-Kolehmainen MA. Influence of age, ethnicity and sex on body composition thresholds for the accumulation of visceral adipose tissue in adults. American Journal of Sports Science. 2019;**7**(3):111-120

[62] CCC C, Faucher P, Czernichow S, Oppert J-M. Obesidad del adulto. Tratado de Medicina. 2017;**21**(2):1-10

[63] Izaola O et al. Inflammation and obesity (lipoinflammation). Nutrición Hospitalaria. 2015;**31**(6):2352-2358

[64] Bluher M. Clinical relevance of adipokines. Diabetes and Metabolism Journal. 2012;**36**(5):317-327

[65] Cremona A et al. Effect of exercise modality on markers of insulin sensitivity and blood glucose control in pregnancies complicated with gestational diabetes mellitus: A systematic review. Obesity Science and Practice. 2018;**4**(5):455-467

[66] Makki K, Froguel P, Wolowczuk I. Adipose tissue in obesity-related inflammation and insulin resistance: Cells, cytokines, and chemokines. ISRN Inflammation. 2013;**2013**:139239

[67] Mancuso P. The role of adipokines in chronic inflammation. ImmunoTargets and Therapy. 2016;**5**:47-56

[68] Grigoras A et al. Perivascular adipose tissue in cardiovascular diseases-an update. Anatolian Journal of Cardiology. 2019;**22**(5):219-231

[69] Parisi L, Gini E. Macrophage polarization in chronic inflammatory diseases: Killers or builders? Journal of Immunology Research. 2018;**2018**:8917804

[70] Marie C et al. Regulation by anti-inflammatory cytokines (IL-4, IL-10, IL-13, TGFbeta) of interleukin-8 production by LPS- and/ or TNFalpha-activated human polymorphonuclear cells. Mediators of Inflammation. 1996;**5**(5):334-340

[71] Calder PC. Omega-3 fatty acids and inflammatory processes: From molecules to man. Biochemical Society Transactions. 2017;**45**(5):1105-1115

[72] Ieronymaki E et al. Insulin signaling and insulin resistance facilitate trained immunity in macrophages through metabolic and epigenetic changes. Frontiers in Immunology. 2019;**10**:1330

[73] Unamuno X et al. Adipokine dysregulation and adipose tissue inflammation in human obesity. European Journal of Clinical Investigation. 2018;**48**(9):e12997

[74] Gregoire FM, Smas CM, Sul HS. Understanding adipocyte differentiation. Physiological Reviews. 1998;**78**(3):783-809

[75] Park A, Kim WK, Bae KH. Distinction of white, beige and brown adipocytes derived from mesenchymal stem cells. World Journal of Stem Cells. 2014;**6**(1):33-42

[76] Lefterova MI et al. PPARgamma and the global map of adipogenesis and beyond. Trends in Endocrinology and Metabolism. 2014;**25**(6):293-302

[77] Lin FT, Lane MD. CCAAT/enhancer binding protein alpha is sufficient to initiate the 3T3-L1 adipocyte differentiation program. Proceedings of the National Academy of Sciences of the United States of America. 1994;**91**(19):8757-8761

[78] Guo L, Li X, Tang QQ. Transcriptional regulation of adipocyte differentiation: A central role for CCAAT/enhancer-binding protein (C/EBP) beta. The Journal of Biological Chemistry. 2015;**290**(2):755-761

[79] Grundy SM. Adipose tissue and metabolic syndrome: Too much, too little or neither. European Journal of Clinical Investigation. 2015;**45**(11):1209-1217

[80] Moseti D, Regassa A, Kim WK. Molecular regulation of adipogenesis and potential anti-adipogenic bioactive molecules. International Journal of Molecular Sciences. 2016;**17**(1):124

[81] Trayhurn P, Drevon CA, Eckel J. Secreted proteins from adipose tissue and skeletal muscle—Adipokines, myokines and adipose/muscle cross-talk. Archives of Physiology and Biochemistry. 2011;**117**(2):47-56

[82] Raschke S, Eckel J. Adipo-myokines: Two sides of the same coin-mediators of inflammation and mediators of exercise. Mediators of Inflammation. 2013;**2013**:320724

[83] Li F et al. Myokines and adipokines: Involvement in the crosstalk between skeletal muscle and adipose tissue. Cytokine & Growth Factor Reviews. 2017;**33**:73-82

[84] Rodriguez A et al. Crosstalk between adipokines and myokines in fat browning. Acta Physiologica (Oxford, England). 2017;**219**(2):362-381

[85] Sahin-Efe A et al. Irisin and leptin concentrations in relation to obesity, and developing type 2 diabetes: A cross sectional and a prospective case-control study nested in the normative aging study. Metabolism. 2018;**79**:24-32

[86] Ye X et al. Irisin reverses insulin resistance in C2C12 cells via the p38-MAPK-PGC-1alpha pathway. Peptides. 2019;**119**:170120

[87] Meijer K et al. Human primary adipocytes exhibit immune cell function: Adipocytes prime inflammation independent of macrophages. PLoS One. 2011;**6**(3):e17154

[88] Sell H et al. Skeletal muscle insulin resistance induced by adipocyte-conditioned medium: Underlying mechanisms and reversibility. American Journal of Physiology. Endocrinology and Metabolism. 2008;**294**(6):E1070-E1077

[89] Sell H et al. Monocyte chemotactic protein-1 is a potential player in the negative cross-talk between adipose tissue and skeletal muscle. Endocrinology. 2006;**147**(5):2458-2467

[90] Lobo SM et al. TNF-alpha modulates statin effects on secretion and expression of MCP-1, PAI-1 and adiponectin in 3T3-L1 differentiated adipocytes. Cytokine. 2012;**60**(1):150-156

[91] Famulla S et al. Pigment epithelium-derived factor (PEDF) is one of the most abundant proteins secreted by human adipocytes and induces insulin resistance and inflammatory

signaling in muscle and fat cells. International Journal of Obesity. 2011;**35**(6):762-772

[92] Fisher FM et al. FGF21 regulates PGC-1alpha and browning of white adipose tissues in adaptive thermogenesis. Genes & Development. 2012;**26**(3):271-281

[93] Wu Y, Zhou S, Smas CM. Downregulated expression of the secreted glycoprotein follistatin-like 1 (Fstl1) is a robust hallmark of preadipocyte to adipocyte conversion. Mechanisms of Development. 2010;**127**(3-4):183-202

[94] Rudrapatna S et al. Obesity and muscle-macrophage crosstalk in humans and mice: A systematic review. Obesity Reviews. 2019;**20**(11):1572-1596

[95] Landrier JF, Derghal A, Mounien L. MicroRNAs in obesity and related metabolic disorders. Cell. 2019;**8**(8):859

[96] Naukkarinen J et al. Causes and consequences of obesity: The contribution of recent twin studies. International Journal of Obesity. 2012;**36**(8):1017-1024

[97] Xia Q, Grant SF. The genetics of human obesity. Annals of the New York Academy of Sciences. 2013;**1281**:178-190

[98] de Luca C, Olefsky JM. Inflammation and insulin resistance. FEBS Letters. 2008;**582**(1):97-105

[99] Ota T. Chemokine systems link obesity to insulin resistance. Diabetes and Metabolism Journal. 2013;**37**(3):165-172

[100] Bourlier V, Bouloumie A. Role of macrophage tissue infiltration in obesity and insulin resistance. Diabetes & Metabolism. 2009;**35**(4):251-260

[101] Wang Z, Nakayama T. Inflammation, a link between obesity and cardiovascular disease. Mediators of Inflammation. 2010;**2010**:535918

[102] Chawla A, Nguyen KD, Goh YP. Macrophage-mediated inflammation in metabolic disease. Nature Reviews. Immunology. 2011;**11**(11):738-749

[103] Ouchi N et al. Adipokines in inflammation and metabolic disease. Nature Reviews. Immunology. 2011;**11**(2):85-97

[104] McNelis JC, Olefsky JM. Macrophages, immunity, and metabolic disease. Immunity. 2014;**41**(1):36-48

[105] Schipper HS et al. Adipose tissue-resident immune cells: Key players in immunometabolism. Trends in Endocrinology and Metabolism. 2012;**23**(8):407-415

[106] Yao L et al. Roles of the chemokine system in development of obesity, insulin resistance, and cardiovascular disease. Journal of Immunology Research. 2014;**2014**:181450

[107] Poon AK et al. Short-term repeatability of insulin resistance indexes in older adults: The atherosclerosis risk in communities study. The Journal of Clinical Endocrinology and Metabolism. 2018;**103**(6):2175-2181

[108] Samuel VT, Shulman GI. Mechanisms for insulin resistance: Common threads and missing links. Cell. 2012;**148**(5):852-871

[109] Chakraborty C et al. Influence of miRNA in insulin signaling pathway and insulin resistance: Micro-molecules with a major role in type-2 diabetes. Wiley Interdisciplinary Reviews: RNA. 2014;**5**(5):697-712

[110] Zhang J, Li S, Li L, Li M, Guo C, Yao J, et al. Exosome and exosomal microRNA: Trafficking, sorting, and function. Genomics Proteomics Bioinformatics. 2015;**13**(1):17-24

[111] Ness-Abramof R, Apovian CM. Waist circumference measurement in clinical practice. Nutrition in Clinical Practice. 2008;**23**(4):397-404

[112] Khoury S, Tran N. Circulating microRNAs: Potential biomarkers for common malignancies. Biomarkers in Medicine. 2015;**9**(2):131-151

[113] van Rooij E. The art of microRNA research. Circulation Research. 2011;**108**(2):219-234

[114] Lagarrigue S et al. CDK4 is an essential insulin effector in adipocytes. The Journal of Clinical Investigation. 2016;**126**(1):335-348

[115] Di Meo S, Iossa S, Venditti P. Skeletal muscle insulin resistance: Role of mitochondria and other ROS sources. The Journal of Endocrinology. 2017;**233**(1):R15-r42

[116] Edgerton DS et al. Effects of insulin on the metabolic control of hepatic gluconeogenesis in vivo. Diabetes. 2009;**58**(12):2766-2775

[117] Miyake K et al. Hyperinsulinemia, glucose intolerance, and dyslipidemia induced by acute inhibition of phosphoinositide 3-kinase signaling in the liver. The Journal of Clinical Investigation. 2002;**110**(10):1483-1491

[118] Inoue H et al. Role of hepatic STAT3 in brain-insulin action on hepatic glucose production. Cell Metabolism. 2006;**3**(4):267-275

[119] Pocai A et al. Hypothalamic K(ATP) channels control hepatic glucose production. Nature. 2005;**434**(7036):1026-1031

[120] Yu C et al. Mechanism by which fatty acids inhibit insulin activation of insulin receptor substrate-1 (IRS-1)-associated phosphatidylinositol 3-kinase activity in muscle. The Journal of Biological Chemistry. 2002;**277**(52):50230-50236

[121] Cherrington AD. The role of hepatic insulin receptors in the regulation of glucose production. The Journal of Clinical Investigation. 2005;**115**(5):1136-1139

[122] Ferrannini E et al. Effect of fatty acids on glucose production and utilization in man. The Journal of Clinical Investigation. 1983;**72**(5):1737-1747

[123] Perry RJ et al. Hepatic acetyl CoA links adipose tissue inflammation to hepatic insulin resistance and type 2 diabetes. Cell. 2015;**160**(4):745-758

[124] Gupta MK, Vasudevan NT. GPCRs and insulin receptor signaling in conversation: Novel avenues for drug discovery. Current Topics in Medicinal Chemistry. 2019;**19**(16):1436-1444

[125] Chen L et al. Acetyl-CoA carboxylase (ACC) as a therapeutic target for metabolic syndrome and recent developments in ACC1/2 inhibitors. Expert Opinion on Investigational Drugs. 2019;**28**(10):917-930

[126] Haeusler RA et al. Integrated control of hepatic lipogenesis versus glucose production requires FoxO transcription factors. Nature Communications. 2014;**5**:5190

[127] Perry RJ et al. Mechanisms by which a very-low-calorie diet reverses hyperglycemia in a rat model of type 2 diabetes. Cell Metabolism. 2018;**27**(1):210-217.e3

[128] Ferrannini E. Insulin resistance versus insulin deficiency in non-insulin-dependent diabetes mellitus: Problems and prospects. Endocrine Reviews. 1998;**19**(4):477-490

[129] Taniguchi CM, Emanuelli B, Kahn CR. Critical nodes in signalling pathways: Insights into insulin action. Nature Reviews. Molecular Cell Biology. 2006;**7**(2):85-96

[130] Savage DB, Petersen KF, Shulman GI. Disordered lipid metabolism and the pathogenesis of insulin resistance. Physiological Reviews. 2007;**87**(2):507-520

[131] Dresner A et al. Effects of free fatty acids on glucose transport and IRS-1-associated phosphatidylinositol 3-kinase activity. The Journal of Clinical Investigation. 1999;**103**(2):253-259

[132] Hotamisligil GS et al. IRS-1-mediated inhibition of insulin receptor tyrosine kinase activity in TNF-alpha- and obesity-induced insulin resistance. Science. 1996;**271**(5249):665-668

[133] Boura-Halfon S, Zick Y. Phosphorylation of IRS proteins, insulin action, and insulin resistance. American Journal of Physiology. Endocrinology and Metabolism. 2009;**296**(4):E581-E591

[134] Houstis N, Rosen ED, Lander ES. Reactive oxygen species have a causal role in multiple forms of insulin resistance. Nature. 2006;**440**(7086):944-948

[135] Muoio DM, Neufer PD. Lipid-induced mitochondrial stress and insulin action in muscle. Cell Metabolism. 2012;**15**(5):595-605

[136] Altintas MM et al. Mast cells, macrophages, and crown-like structures distinguish subcutaneous from visceral fat in mice. Journal of Lipid Research. 2011;**52**(3):480-488

[137] De Lorenzo A et al. New obesity classification criteria as a tool for bariatric surgery indication. World Journal of Gastroenterology. 2016;**22**(2):681-703

[138] Stefan N, Schick F, Haring HU. Causes, characteristics, and consequences of metabolically unhealthy normal weight in humans. Cell Metabolism. 2017;**26**(2):292-300

[139] van Vliet-Ostaptchouk JV et al. The prevalence of metabolic syndrome and metabolically healthy obesity in Europe: A collaborative analysis of ten large cohort studies. BMC Endocrine Disorders. 2014;**14**:9

[140] Crewe C, An YA, Scherer PE. The ominous triad of adipose tissue dysfunction: Inflammation, fibrosis, and impaired angiogenesis. The Journal of Clinical Investigation. 2017;**127**(1):74-82

[141] Bluher M. Adipose tissue dysfunction contributes to obesity related metabolic diseases. Best Practice & Research. Clinical Endocrinology & Metabolism. 2013;**27**(2):163-177

[142] Woo CY et al. Mitochondrial dysfunction in adipocytes as a primary cause of adipose tissue inflammation. Diabetes & Metabolism Journal. 2019;**43**(3):247-256

[143] Chylikova J et al. M1/M2 macrophage polarization in human obese adipose tissue. Biomedical Papers of the Medical Faculty of the University Palacky, Olomouc, Czech Republic. 2018;**162**(2):79-82

[144] Kratz M et al. Metabolic dysfunction drives a mechanistically distinct proinflammatory phenotype in adipose tissue macrophages. Cell Metabolism. 2014;**20**(4):614-625

[145] Mori S et al. Characteristic expression of extracellular matrix in subcutaneous adipose tissue development and adipogenesis; comparison with visceral adipose tissue. International Journal of Biological Sciences. 2014;**10**(8):825-833

[146] Engin AB. Adipocyte-macrophage cross-talk in obesity. Advances in Experimental Medicine and Biology. 2017;**960**:327-343

[147] Karczewski J et al. Obesity and inflammation. European Cytokine Network. 2018;**29**(3):83-94

[148] Fang Z, Pyne S, Pyne NJ. Ceramide and sphingosine 1-phosphate in adipose dysfunction. Progress in Lipid Research. 2019;**74**:145-159

[149] Godsland IF. Insulin resistance and hyperinsulinaemia in the development and progression of cancer. Clinical Science (London, England). 2009;**118**(5):315-332

Chapter 3

Obesity as a Promoter of Cancer Development and Progression

Nicole Bonan and Katie DeCicco-Skinner

Abstract

The incidence of obesity is growing worldwide. In the United States, it is now estimated that one in three adults is categorized as obese. Obesity is a risk factor for multiple forms of cancer, and obese individuals have a higher risk of death. This chapter will share insight into how obesity is associated with cancer development, progression, and drug resistance by looking at the interplay between adipocytes (fat cells) and cancer cells. In particular, we will focus on alterations that occur in an obese state and biological mechanisms such as inflammation, oxidative stress, and hormonal imbalances that contribute to increased cancer risk.

Keywords: adipocyte, adipokine, adiponectin, adipose, cancer, estrogen, HIF, hormone, hyperinsulinemia, hypoxia, IFNγ, inflammation, insulin, leptin, MAPK, obesity, resistance, T cell

1. Introduction

Obesity has reached epidemic levels in the United States, and it is a growing health concern worldwide. It is estimated that one in three adults in the US is obese, while another one in three is overweight [1]. Worldwide, obesity has close to tripled since 1975. In 2016, 13% of adults were categorized as obese and 39% as overweight [2]. Obesity is a risk factor for multiple diseases, including heart disease, stroke, type 2 diabetes, and cancer, and obese individuals have a higher risk of death [1–3]. In the US, quality-adjusted life years lost to obesity are now higher than those lost to smoking [4].

"Obesity" is most often defined by body mass index (BMI), a calculation based on a ratio of one's height and weight (kg/m^2). "Obese" refers to a BMI of 30 or more, while "overweight" is categorized as a BMI between 25–30 and "normal weight" is defined as a BMI of 18.5–25.

Cancer describes the uncontrolled growth of cells which can metastasize, or spread, to other parts of the body. It can occur in any tissue and can be caused by a variety of environmental and genetic factors. About 15–20% of all cancers are estimated to be caused by being obese or overweight [5, 6]. Obese patients diagnosed with many types of cancers tend to have a worse prognosis, increased risk of metastatic cancers, and a shorter remission period than normal weight individuals [4, 7]. However, some cancers are more strongly associated with obesity than others [4, 7], and the correlation is dependent mainly on tissue type and patient cohort [5]. Cancers that are most closely correlated with obesity include: kidney [8], endometrial [9], ovarian [8], liver [10], pancreatic [11], gastrointestinal [8], colorectal [12], prostate [13], and postmenopausal breast cancer [14]; and multiple myeloma [7, 8, 15, 16]. Postmenopausal women are an especially susceptible patient cohort, as half of all cancers in this group are caused by

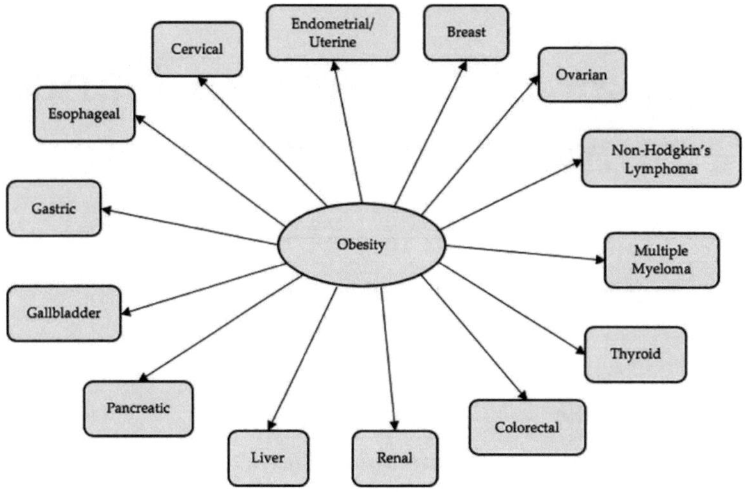

Figure 1.
Obesity can increase the risk of many cancers, including: cervical, endometrial, uterine, breast, ovarian, thyroid, colorectal, renal, liver, pancreatic, gallbladder, gastric, and esophageal cancer; non-Hodgkin's lymphoma; and multiple myeloma.

obesity [5]. The most common cancers caused by obesity in post-menopausal women are breast, endometrial, and ovarian cancers (**Figure 1**).

Besides storing lipids, adipose tissue is increasingly being recognized as the largest endocrine organ in the body. The adipose tissue itself is comprised of multiple cell types, including adipocytes, immune cells, and endothelial cells, among others [17]. Adipocytes themselves can secrete a variety of adipokines, hormones, and inflammatory factors [17]. As such, adipocytes are involved in signaling pathways with neighboring cells. Signaling mechanisms in the adipose tissue are altered by obesity and can contribute to cancer development, progression, and drug resistance. Cancers that are in direct contact with adipocytes, such as breast cancer, and even cancers that are in close proximity to adipocytes, such as colon cancer and endometrial cancer, are most susceptible to increased aggression stimulated by adipocyte signaling [17]. This chapter will focus on a few of the mechanisms through which adipocytes affect the tumor microenvironment (TME), including insulin resistance and hyperinsulinemia, sex steroid hormone signaling, changes in the adipokine profile, and chronic inflammation and hypoxia.

2. Adipose tissue

Generally, adipose tissue is divided into two main groups: visceral adipose tissue (VAT), which surrounds internal organs, and subcutaneous adipose tissue (SAT), which is located just under the skin. These two types of adipose tissue show large differences in metabolic activity and influence on disease risk [18]. Generally, both SAT and VAT increase in volume in obesity. However, too much VAT is associated with more negative health effects than SAT.

Visceral obesity, rather than subcutaneous obesity, increases the risk of multiple diseases including cancer [18]. This phenomenon is manly a result of the differing physiological roles of VAT and SAT. VAT acts as an endocrine organ and can signal other parts of the body via adipokine and cytokine secretion [18]. It also contains more immune cells and is more highly vascularized than SAT [19]. VAT adipocytes are generally more metabolically active than SAT adipocytes [19], and as such, most of the changes that occur to adipose tissue during obesity occur in VAT rather than in SAT [19]. Overall, VAT is a stronger predictor of mortality due to obesity than SAT [19], especially when the VAT surrounding abdominal organs is high [18].

SAT acts as more of a storage tissue than VAT, as SAT adipocytes absorb free fatty acids and store them as triglycerides [19]. Increased SAT is generally not strongly associated with obesity-related cancers [18], with the exception of abdominal SAT. Multiple studies have shown that increased abdominal SAT can promote cancer growth progression, sometimes independently of overall adiposity [15, 20]. SAT (excluding abdominal SAT) has actually shown a somewhat protective role in cancer. Patients with more SAT generally have increased survival rates after treatment than those with less SAT [21].

This paper will focus on VAT, as this tissue type is most strongly correlated with cancer risk. Thus, references made to obesity and adipocytes throughout the rest of this paper refer to VAT.

3. Insulin resistance and hyperinsulinemia

Insulin is a hormone that is primarily responsible for stimulating glucose uptake and storage, but it is involved in multiple evolutionarily conserved pathways involving cell growth and proliferation [22, 23]. This pluripotency is not unusual. Signaling pathways related to nutrient availability and growth are closely related, as uptake of nutrients is essential for supporting growth on both a systemic and intracellular level in the body [24].

Obesity, which is characterized by an excess of nutrient availability, stimulates the body to increase insulin secretion and continually activate growth pathways. In this way, obesity can change the balance of inter- and intracellular signaling that controls cycle progression, growth, proliferation, and angiogenesis. Any of these effects in excess can contribute to neoplastic transformation, and since these pathways are highly conserved and interconnected, any alterations to one pathway risk overcompensation through another [24]. Thus, the increase in insulin secretion and growth activation caused by obesity can directly contribute to tumor development and progression.

3.1 Insulin and insulin-like growth factors

Insulin is secreted by pancreatic beta cells when serum glucose levels are elevated. The insulin then enters the bloodstream and binds insulin receptors (IR) on the plasma membrane of target cells. IRs are a type of receptor tyrosine kinase (RTK). Thus, binding of the ligand causes autophosphorylation of the tyrosine residues on the cytoplasmic tails of IRs, activating signaling pathways related to cell growth, proliferation, and glucose metabolism [5, 24, 25] (**Figure 2**).

There are two isoforms of IRs that are created by alternative splicing of the insulin receptor (INSR) gene: IR-B and IR-A. IR-B is expressed at high levels in adipocytes, hepatocytes, and muscle cells, as it is the isoform that regulates glucose metabolism [26]. IR-A is usually expressed at low levels in most normal cells compared to IR-B, but it is the isoform that is often over-expressed in cancer cells [26].

Insulin-like growth factors (IGFs) are endocrine hormones that are homologous to and have a similar mechanism of action as insulin [24, 27]. While insulin is primarily involved in glucose metabolism via IR/PI3K signaling, IGFs are directly responsible for stimulating cell growth and proliferation via IGF-1 receptor (IGF-1R)/mitogen activated protein kinase (MAPK) signaling (**Figure 2**). However, IR and IGF-1R signaling overlap to a large extent, and the exact conditions that determine their specificity are not well understood [23].

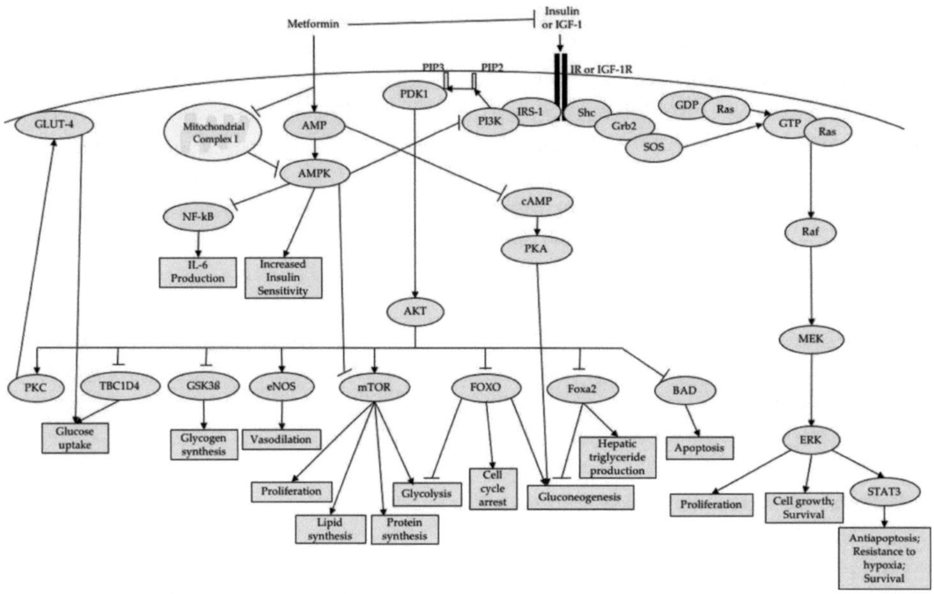

Figure 2.
IR and IGF-1R can activate the same signaling pathways. In normal cells, stimulation of either receptor activates pathways related to cell growth and proliferation. IR is also responsible for regulating glucose metabolism, while IGF-1R activates signaling pathways related to evasion of apoptosis, metastasis, and angiogenesis. In obesity, this specificity is lost. Treatment with metformin activates AMPK signaling, which blocks many of the pathways activated by AKT and can decrease tumor growth and progression.

There are two main types of IGFs, IGF-I and IGF-II, both of which are secreted by the liver in response to other growth hormones [5, 24]. Once in the tissue and bloodstream, IGFs are generally bound by IGF binding proteins (IGFBP), which both increase the half-life of IGFs [27] and prevent them from binding receptors [24, 27]. When serum glucose levels are elevated, IGFs dissociate from their binding proteins. IGF-1 can then bind IGF-1 receptor (IGF-1R), an RTK that is similar to IR [24], or, with lower affinity, IR-A [23]. Binding of IGF-1 to its receptor can activate MAPK signaling, inhibit p53, or stimulate hypoxia-inducible factor 1 alpha (HIF-1α) expression. The result of these pathways are cell growth and proliferation, evasion of apoptosis and metastasis, and angiogenesis, respectively [5]. IGF-II can bind both IGF-1R and IR-A with high affinity [5] and IR-B with low affinity [23].

Insulin and IGF signaling pathways are highly conserved, as they are essential for normal development [24, 27]. As such, disruptions in the balance of signaling through these pathways, such as changes in metabolism associated with obesity, can lead to cancer development and progression.

3.2 Insulin resistance, hyperinsulinemia, and cancer

In obese individuals, glucose is constantly produced in the liver in response to nutrient excess, and adipose tissue over-secretes insulin in response. However, chronic over-secretion of insulin can lead to insulin resistance. This condition occurs when the body only minimally responds to insulin and thus cannot metabolize glucose. To compensate, beta cells secrete even more insulin, causing hyperinsulinemia [5]. The high serum insulin levels caused by hyperinsulinemia have multiple physiological effects that can contribute to cancer progression.

High serum insulin levels can increase production of IGF-1, which, as discussed earlier, activates signaling pathways related to growth, proliferation, evasion of apoptosis and metastasis, and angiogenesis [5]. Cancer cells can then use these pathways to meet their high metabolic demands [24]. Insulin can stimulate production of growth hormone receptor (GHR), which, when bound to its ligand, stimulates hepatic synthesis of IGF-1 [5]. Insulin can also decrease production of IGFBP-1 and 2. This decrease leads to an increase in free IGF-1 in the serum [5].

Increased insulin and IGF-1 serum levels can cause overproduction and overstimulation of IR-A and IGF-1R, which is a phenomenon that is commonly observed in cancer cells [23]. The signaling pathways activated by IR and IGF-1R overlap, so overstimulation of both receptors leads to amplification of shared pathways such as mTOR and MAPK. As a result, excessive cell growth and proliferation can be stimulated [23]. The specific functions of insulin, IGFs, IR, and IGF-1R also often become convoluted in the context of cancer. In normal cells, IR is mainly responsible for controlling metabolism, while IGF-1R is more involved in regulating cell growth [23]. However, because IR and IGF-1R are highly homologous, a hybrid of the two receptors can form when they are both overexpressed. The hybrid has a higher affinity for IGF-1 than for insulin, which amplifies IGF signaling and thus contributes to cell growth, proliferation, and evasion of apoptosis. This hybrid can be expressed in normal cells, but it tends to be expressed more highly in cancer cells, especially of the breast and thyroid [5].

Some cancer treatments target IGF-1R, as this receptor is more historically known for its role in regulating cell growth. However, while preclinical studies targeting this receptor were promising, clinical studies were widely unsuccessful, and many were terminated [23, 28]. Moreover, sensitivity to IGF-1R inhibition varies widely among tumors even though most have an overexpression of IGF-1R [23, 28, 29]. Current studies are focusing on finding biomarkers that can predict sensitivity to IGF-1R inhibition [28]. Other studies aim to determine whether combination therapy might make IGF-1R inhibition more viable, such as IGF-1R inhibitors given with mTOR or IR inhibitors [28]. Since the functions of IGF-1R and IR overlap in the context of cancer, signaling through IR may be a mechanism of resistance to IGF-1R inhibitors. Some studies are researching whether targeting both IGF-1R and IR can prevent resistance from developing to IGF-1R inhibitors [23].

Other studies aim to determine whether common drugs used to treat diabetes, such as metformin, can have anti-cancer effects. So far, these studies have shown promising results. Metformin is used to decrease serum levels of insulin and hepatic glucose production in diabetic patients. However, metformin has been found to also increase AMPK production via inhibition of mitochondrial complex I. AMPK can then increase in insulin sensitivity and inhibit the mTOR/AKT pathway, which decreases glycolysis and lipid synthesis [30] (**Figure 2**). Both animal and clinical studies thus far have shown that metformin can decrease the risk of tumor development and progression, though the exact mechanisms of action of the drug have yet to be elucidated [23]. The main side effect of the drug is gastrointestinal disturbance, which occurs in about 30% of patients [30].

In summary, hyperinsulinemia is a common condition in obesity that is characterized by over-secretion of insulin and IGF-1. Both of these factors can contribute to overexpression of IR, IGF-1R, and the IR-A/IGF-1R hybrid, which can dysregulate growth and metabolism and have tumor-promoting effects.

4. Sex steroid hormones

It is already well-established that obesity can directly increase the concentration of circulating sex steroid hormones (SSH), especially estrogen. As such, obesity is a known risk factor for cancers that can be caused in part by increased levels of these hormones, such as breast, endometrial, uterine, ovarian, and prostate cancers [5, 6, 24].

Estrogen is formed from the aromatization of androgens such as testosterone and androstenedione [24]. In premenopausal women, this aromatization takes place mainly in the ovaries [24], but it shifts to the adipose tissue and epidermis in postmenopausal women [17]. Estrogen production occurs primarily in the testes of men [31]. Once in circulation, estrogen can have multiple physiological effects.

Estrogen can bind ERs on cells to stimulate cell division [4], cell cycle progression [32], and increase proliferation and angiogenesis [24]. ER activation is a major contributor to cancer progression in ER+ breast cancers. ER+ breast cancers account for approximately 70% of human breast cancers overall [33], and obesity is known to increase the risk of these cancers in postmenopausal women [34]. In these cancers, overactive ER signaling can cause DNA damage by dysregulating genes that control cell cycle, such as Cyclin D1. Overactive ER signaling can also increase the formation of R-loops in genes that are activated by estrogen. R-loops are formed when newly-synthesized RNA binds its DNA template, and they can regulate certain aspects of transcription. However, in the context of ER overstimulation, an excess of R-loops can lead to double-stranded breaks in genes activated by estrogen, contributing to genome instability and dysregulation of cell growth and proliferation [32, 35]. Hormone therapy is often given post-surgery in ER+ breast cancers, which has been shown to improve survival and decrease the risk of relapse [33], illustrating the large extent to which ER signaling contributes to cancer progression.

The increased levels of estrogen caused by obesity can also increase IR-A expression and amplify IGF signaling in breast cancer. These factors can contribute to IGF-1R inhibitor resistance and inhibition of apoptosis, respectively, as discussed in the previous section [4, 5]. In addition, estrogen can act as a mitogen, activating MAPK pathways and RTKs that, like ER, lead to cell cycle progression, proliferation, and survival [5].

There are a few mechanisms that control the increase in circulating SSH caused by obesity. Adipose tissue can produce aromatase, and increased adiposity is correlated with an increased production of the enzyme. Aromatase stimulates the conversion of androgens to estrogens in both men and postmenopausal women. In excess, the enzyme can increase circulating concentrations of the estrogen estradiol, which can cause DNA damage as discussed [4]. This signaling mechanism is a likely explanation for why breast cancer risk increases with BMI in postmenopausal women that do not receive hormone replacement therapy [24]. Adipose tissue can also decrease production of globulins, which would otherwise bind and inhibit the activity of hormones such as estradiol [24], contributing to DNA damage.

Severe obesity can also modulate other molecules that can contribute to cancer risk and progression. The concentration of circulating glucocorticoids, hormones that act to negatively regulate cell cycle and decrease inflammation, can be downregulated [24]. Severe obesity can also stimulate an increase in serum concentrations of IGF-1 and the pro-inflammatory cytokine IL-6. Both of these molecules can activate the androgen receptor and contribute to survival and proliferation in prostate cancer [24].

5. Adipokines

Adipokines are cytokines that are secreted by adipose tissue. These adipokines can play important roles in metabolism, endocrine activities, satiety, and inflammation [5, 17, 24]. However, adipokines can also both contribute to and suppress tumorigenesis. Obesity is generally correlated with a decrease in tumor-suppressing and an increase in tumor-promoting adipokines. There are multiple types of adipokines, but the most well-researched and abundant adipokines in the human body are leptin and adiponectin [5].

5.1 Leptin

Leptin is the most well-known adipokine, and its main function is to suppress appetite [24]. It is secreted by adipose tissue in response to nutrient availability, and it binds leptin receptors on cells such as neurons, skeletal muscle cells, adipocytes, and epithelial cells [26]. This binding signals a decrease in appetite and creates a negative feedback loop between adipose tissue and the central nervous system [24].

Leptin production increases proportionally with body fat. However, leptin resistance often develops in the context of obesity. This resistance occurs because the adipose tissue in obese patients produces excessive amounts of leptin, which overstimulates leptin receptors. The receptors then become less sensitive to the adipokine, and in response, the adipose tissue secretes even more leptin [26, 36]. As a result, obese patients often experience a dysregulation in appetite where they do not feel satiated even when their body has taken in all necessary nutrients because their bodies do not respond to leptin.

Leptin has other important physiological functions besides appetite suppression. When bound to their ligand, leptin receptors can activate the PI3K, MAPK, and JAK/STAT signaling pathways. All of these pathways lead to either inflammation, cell growth and proliferation, angiogenesis, or prevention of apoptosis [5, 24]. Since leptin is often over-secreted in obesity, this adipokine is known to contribute to the systemic inflammation observed in many obese patients [17, 24, 26], which will be discussed in later sections of this chapter.

Leptin is also a likely link between obesity and cancer. Most studies researching leptin and cancer have been done in a breast cancer model. These studies have found that leptin increases aromatase expression, which upregulates estrogen production and ER signaling [5]. As discussed previously, ER signaling stimulates cell division, proliferation, and angiogenesis, and it prevents apoptosis [4, 24], all of which can contribute to tumorigenesis and cancer progression. Other studies have found that leptin may activate proliferation and survival of cancer cells in *in vitro* models of prostate, endometrium, and colon cancer [24].

5.2 Adiponectin

Adiponectin is the most abundant cytokine in the body, and it is the main hormone produced by adipose tissue [7]. The major roles of adiponectin are to increase sensitivity to insulin [7] and increase energy expenditure [26]. By increasing insulin sensitivity, adiponectin can help prevent the development of insulin resistance and thus can help control glucose metabolism and growth [37]. Adiponectin can also inhibit angiogenesis and migration [37], stimulate apoptosis [24], and downregulate vascular endothelial adhesion molecules and decrease inflammation [37].

Adiponectin has a protective role in carcinogenesis [37], but serum levels of adiponectin tend to decrease with increased BMI and visceral adiposity [26]. Adiponectin activates the AMPK pathway, which can inhibit mTOR and cause cell cycle arrest [37]. It also inactivates MAPK1/3 and ERK1/2 and can stimulate apoptosis by inducing expression of p53 and Bax and decreasing expression of Bcl-2 [5]. However, estrogen and insulin both can suppress adiponectin secretion [5]. Thus, there is a complex balance of sex hormones, insulin, and adipokines that contribute to both obesity and cancer.

Current studies have shown the beneficial effects of adiponectin in cancer. Breast cancer risk is lower when serum levels of adiponectin are elevated in both pre and postmenopausal women [5]. Similarly, increased levels of adiponectin are associated with decreased risk of endometrial, colon, and prostate cancers [4]. Adiponectin has also been shown to inhibit growth in *in vivo* models of all of these cancers [24]. Lower levels of adiponectin in men are correlated with a higher risk of colon cancer [5], and adiponectin has been shown to suppress the formation of colon polyps in mouse models of colon cancer [26]. In general, increased levels of adiponectin are correlated with a decrease in both the occurrence and severity of multiple cancers [5].

Other adipokines besides leptin and adiponectin exist. Resistin may be involved in promoting inflammation and angiogenesis, which can contribute to tumorigenesis [4]. Plasminogen activator inhibitor type 1 (PAI-1) is generally used as an indicator of poor prognosis in breast cancer, especially in obese women [5]. High levels of PAI-1 often indicate low peroxisome proliferator-activated receptor gamma (PPARγ) function, which is a receptor that induces apoptosis and decreases proliferation. However, PPARγ expression is often downregulated in obesity. PAI-1 can also inhibit apoptosis and induce inflammation, neutrophil recruitment, proliferation of smooth muscle cells, cell adhesion, and migration, all of which can contribute to tumorigenesis [5]. Growth-regulated oncogene alpha (GRO-α), tissue inhibitor of metalloproteinases 1 (TIMP-1), and thrombopoietin (TPO) are adipokines that tend to be over-secreted in obesity and are believed to promote carcinogenesis. GRO-α can promote inflammation and tumorigenesis; GRO-α and TIMP-1 can promote cell proliferation, angiogenesis, and prevent apoptosis; and TPO can stimulate cell proliferation and differentiation of megakaryocytes [5].

6. Inflammation and hypoxia

The chronic nutrient overload that is characteristic of obesity contributes to inflammation and hypoxia both in adipose tissue and systemically. These effects can impact the tumor microenvironment (TME) to promote tumorigenesis and cancer progression through a variety of mechanisms.

In general, chronic nutrient overload leads to chronic inflammation of the adipose tissue, which is characterized by a sustained increase in inflammatory cytokines and infiltration of macrophages. Levels of adiponectin decrease, while leptin levels increase [26]. The inflammation can also induce hypoxia in the tissue, which can in turn induce more inflammation. Hypoxia is a state of low oxygen. One of the hallmarks of hypoxia is an increase in production of reactive oxygen species (ROS), which can mutate the DNA of nearby cells. These mutations can give cells a potentially cancerous phenotype. In these ways, chronic inflammation and hypoxia can contribute to tumorigenesis and cancer progression [17].

The TME describes the cellular environment that surrounds and feeds a tumor. Once a tumor is established, cells in the TME begin to behave in ways that promote the growth of the cancer. Normal mechanisms for blocking inflammation and encouraging immune surveillance are lost, and metabolic signaling is altered in order to promote the increased energy demand of rapidly-dividing cancer cells. This section will briefly outline the role of obesity-induced inflammation and hypoxia in carcinogenesis and in the TME overall.

6.1 The role of leptin in inflammation and hypoxia

The most notable effect of chronic inflammation in adipose tissue is an over-secretion of leptin, an adipokine that was discussed previously in this chapter. Leptin can in turn induce more inflammation and hypoxia.

Leptin can stimulate cells in the TME to increase transcription of signaling molecules such as nitric oxide (NO) and cyclooxygenase-2 (COX-2) [17]. NO is synthesized by nitric oxide synthases (NOS). The main role of NO is to respond to infection by causing inflammation and tissue damage. In excess, NO destroys enough tissue to induce a state of hypoxia, which is most often the case in the TME and in obesity. This tissue destruction stimulates more inflammation as a result of innate immune cell activation, further exacerbating the cycle. COX-2 upregulates production of prostaglandins, which are precursors for inflammation, proliferation, and survival. It is downstream of NF-kB, which can be activated by the proinflammatory cytokine IL-1β. Overexpression of COX-2 has been observed in cancers including those of the prostate, colon, breast, lung, cervix, pancreas, skin, intestine, and stomach [38], and increased IL-1β expression in tumor cells is correlated with poor prognosis [17].

Leptin can also stimulate innate immune cells in the TME to secrete proinflammatory cytokines including IL-1, IL-6, TNFα, and IFNγ. IL-1 and IL-6 are used as markers for poor prognosis in many obesity-related cancers. IL-1 can activate NF-kB signaling to stimulate cytokine production and cell survival. IL-1 signaling through NF-kB also upregulates expression of hypoxia inducible factor 1 (HIF-1) in the context of obesity-induced inflammation, which induces hypoxia in the adipose tissue and supports angiogenesis, inflammation, and increased energy metabolism [26]. HIF-1 is correlated with increased metastatic spread and poor prognosis of cancer [5].

IL-6 expression is known to be elevated in obese patients [26]. It induces hypoxia in the adipose tissue, and it also stimulates angiogenesis, proliferation, and survival via the JAK/STAT signaling pathway [17]. Like IL-6, TNFα is commonly over-expressed in obese patients. However, TNFα is involved in all stages of tumorigenesis including cell proliferation, transformation, angiogenesis, invasion, and metastasis of cancer cells. TNFα may also stimulate an increase in ROS, which, as discussed, can cause potentially carcinogenic mutations in nearby cells [26].

The role of IFNγ is closely intertwined with T cell signaling in the adipose tissue. IFNγ stimulates naïve CD4+ T cells to differentiate into the type 1 subset (Th1), and it blocks differentiation into other subsets such as type 2 and type 17 helper T cells (Th2 and Th17, respectively). Th1 cells are effector T cells that stimulate macrophages to phagocytose foreign microbes in the body, and they both secrete and are stimulated by IFNγ [39]. Thus, a positive feedback loop occurs in obesity where over-secretion of leptin promotes IFNγ secretion, which stimulates Th1 differentiation, which increases IFNγ secretion. IFNγ can then induce polarization of adipose tissue macrophages (ATMs) to the classical, or M1, phenotype. ATMs are innate immune cells that reside in the adipose tissue, and they are mainly responsible for clearing dead cells and debris [40]. Under normal conditions, the M1 phenotype generally induces an anti-microbial response [41]. It predominates in obese patients, and when activated, M1 ATMs secrete proinflammatory cytokines such as TNFα and IL-6. These cytokines can increase NO concentration in the adipose tissue and contribute to adipose tissue hypoxia. The overall result of M1 ATMs in obese patients is insulin resistance, inflammation, and hypoxia-induced tissue damage [26] (**Figure 3**).

The alternative, or M2, phenotype of ATMs generally induces immune tolerance and tissue remodeling under normal conditions [41]. It predominates in lean patients. These ATMs repair damaged tissue, prevent inflammation from starting, and inhibit insulin resistance. M2 ATMs are activated by anti-inflammatory cytokines secreted by CD4+ type 2 helper T cells (Th2), which include IL-4, IL-10, and IL-13 [26] (**Figure 3**). Since M2 polarization is blocked by IFNγ, levels of M2 ATMs tend to be reduced in obese patients [17].

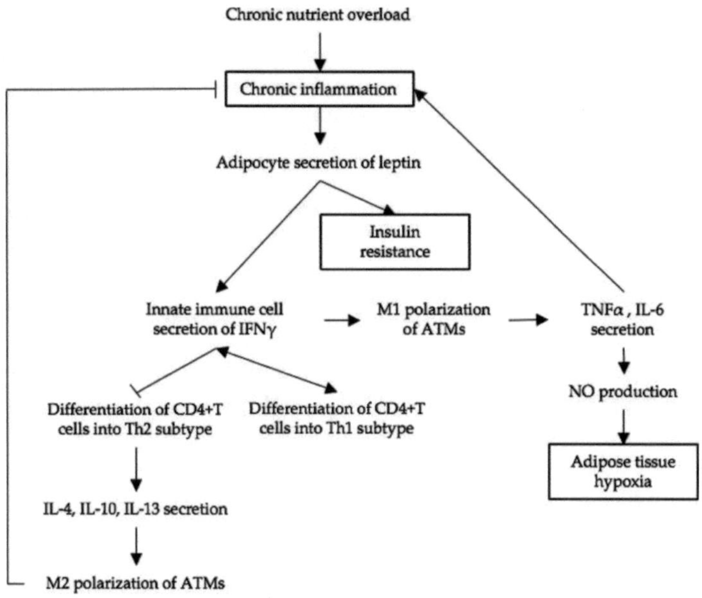

Figure 3.
Chronic nutrient overload, which is characteristic of obesity, can lead to chronic inflammation in the adipose tissue. This inflammation upregulates leptin secretion by adipocytes, which stimulates insulin resistance and IFNγ secretion by innate immune cells. IFNγ blocks differentiation of CD4+ T cells into the Th2 subtype, which would otherwise secrete anti-inflammatory cytokines, induce M2 polarization of ATMs, and block chronic inflammation. Instead, IFNγ stimulates differentiation of CD4+ T cells into the Th1 subtype, which secretes more IFNγ and induces M1 polarization of ATMs. These ATMs secrete more TNFα and IL-6, which contributes to adipose tissue hypoxia, chronic inflammation, and insulin resistance.

6.2 The role of adipocytes in the tumor microenvironment (TME)

Cells and signaling pathways in the TME are altered by the tumor itself in order to promote cancer growth. Generally, the TME is characterized by an increase in inflammation and a decrease in immune surveillance. Adipocytes play a central role in these processes as they are on the interface of cell metabolism and the body's immune response to the tumor. However, the role of adipocytes in the TME is still poorly understood as adipocytes were only recently recognized to have functions besides energy storage.

In direct contrast to the macrophage profile seen in obese patients, M2 macrophages in the TME exist in much higher numbers than their M1 counterparts. Tumor associated adipocytes (TAA), which are adipocytes that are in close proximity to and signal tumor cells, can induce M2 polarization [41]. The macrophages can also be repolarized, or the tumor can recruit M2 macrophages. In the TME, M2 macrophages promote tumor progression via angiogenesis, tissue repair, and secretion of anti-inflammatory cytokines. These cytokines can induce differentiation of T cells into regulatory T cells (Tregs), which prevent the host from mounting an immune response to the tumor. M1 macrophages inhibit tumorigenesis as they can recognize tumor cells as they would a foreign microbe. The M1 macrophages can then phagocytose the tumor cells or release toxins to destroy them. Thus, while M1 macrophages predominate in the adipose tissue of obese patients, the TME induces an increase in M2 polarization. In this way, the ATM profile in obesity may contribute to the inflammation needed to promote the early stages of tumor formation. In later stages, the TME flips the M1:M2 ratio in order to suppress the host's immune response [41].

One of the characteristics of obesity is increased adipocyte death. If this increase in adipocyte cell death occurs in close proximity to a tumor, it can help fuel the growing cancer. The presence of dying adipocytes recruits M1 macrophages, which form crown-like structures (CLSs) around the cells to eliminate them [41]. The CLSs cause a release of DNA from the dying adipocytes into the tissue, which is recognized by toll-like receptor 9 (TLR-9) on macrophages. The macrophages mount a response, recruiting more monocytes to the site of the CLS and inducing more inflammation. The action of CLSs on adipocytes also causes a release of free fatty acids (FFA) into the tissue, which the tumor cells can use for fuel [41].

The "Warburg Effect" describes the change in metabolism from oxidative phosphorylation (OXPHOS) to glycolysis that cancer cells exhibit, and this change may explain some of the immunosuppressive effects of the TME. It is known that the TME has only a small number of effector T cells, which would otherwise detect and eliminate cancer cells. Most cells in the body use OXPHOS for ATP production, but activated CD8+ T cells tend to use glycolysis. Cancer cells also use glycolysis to produce ATP. As a result, cancer cells and effector T cells in the TME compete for the same nutrients. The cancer cells ultimately win, preventing the T cells from meeting their metabolic demands and halting their proliferation near the tumor [42]. Many oncogenes involve activation of glycolytic pathways, while many tumor suppressor genes induce OXPHOS. CD4+ T cells tend to be less affected by the Warburg Effect, however, as they can utilize both glycolysis and OXPHOS to produce ATP. Unstimulated T cells, which do not rapidly divide, use OXPHOS [42].

There are also other mechanisms that contribute to immune suppression in the TME. Tumor cells can stimulate macrophages to produce arginase 1 and the anti-inflammatory cytokines IL-4 and TGFβ. All three factors recruit monocytes to the tumor microenvironment, which in turn recruit tumor-associated macrophages (TAMs). TAMs have multiple effects. They secrete vascular endothelial growth factor (VEGF) and fibroblast growth factor (FGF), which induce angiogenesis and metastasis, respectively. TAMs also block activation of most CD8+ T cells and some CD4+ T cells, which decreases immune surveillance similarly to the Warburg Effect. At the same time, TAMs recruit Tregs to the TME and secrete TGFβ and IL-10, which induce Treg differentiation. The TGFβ can also recruit more monocytes, beginning the cycle again [17].

The presence of Tregs and the decrease in activated T cells play an important role in the ability of the cancer to develop. Tregs are immunosuppressive, and in the context of the tumor microenvironment, they prevent the host from mounting an immune response against the tumor. Interestingly, leptin can both induce and prevent differentiation of T cells into Tregs. IFNγ secretion, stimulated by leptin, can directly block Treg differentiation. However, the proinflammatory cytokines secreted by Th1 T cells, whose differentiation can be induced by leptin, can stimulate tumor cells to secrete C-C motif chemokine 22 (CCL22). This chemokine recruits Tregs to the TME [17, 42, 43]. It is important to note that while Tregs act to suppress the immune system in most cancers, there are some exceptions. Tregs can help slow tumor growth in colorectal cancers, as the Tregs can act to decrease the inflammation needed by the cancer to grow. However, this effect is likely caused by the gut microbiota [44].

The TME can also control adipose-derived stem cell (ASC) activity and fate in order to support cancer growth. ASCs are multipotent stem cells in the adipose tissue. In the context of the TME, ASCs can be induced to secrete matrix metalloproteinases (MMPs). MMPs degrade the extracellular matrix and allow cancer cells access to blood vessels to metastasize to other parts of the body. ASCs can also induce Treg differentiation in a similar manner as TAMs: via TGFβ and IL-10 secretion. Alternatively, the TME can induce ASC differentiation into cancer-associated fibroblast (CAFs) [17], which can then secrete chemokines and growth factors that activate pathways related to cell growth and survival [45].

The TME can also induce hypoxia via anaerobic respiration, even in the presence of oxygen [46]. Under hypoxic conditions, ASCs are recruited to the tissue and are stimulated to secrete VEGF. This allows formation of blood vessels and angiogenesis [17]. Adipocytes can also contribute to angiogenesis in the TME. Adipocytes in obese patients have a higher expression of HIF-1α, which is largely because the adipocytes are rapidly expanding and proliferating in response to nutrient excess. This HIF-1α simulates VEGF secretion. Hypoxia in the adipose tissue also induces IL-6 secretion, which can promote insulin secretion [46].

HIF-1α is a transcription factor that activates hypoxia response elements. In normal conditions, it is hydrolyzed by prolyl hydroxylase domain proteins (PHDs) and ubiquitinated by Von Hippel-Lindau (VHL), which prevents the transcription factor from activating its targets. In hypoxia, however, PHDs and VHL are inhibited. HIF-1α can then bind and activate genes that induce macrophage infiltration and inflammation [46].

HIF-1α can also regulate expression of glycolytic enzymes. This effect is especially important during the metabolic reprogramming that occurs as a result of the Warburg Effect. Most notably, lactate dehydrogenase alpha (LDHα) is transactivated exclusively by HIF-1α. LDHα is responsible for converting pyruvate to lactate during glycolysis in cancer cells [46].

In addition to activating glycolytic pathways, HIF-1α can also block OXPHOS. One of the genes that HIF-1α activates is miR-210, a type of miRNA that is overexpressed in hypoxia in many cancer cells. miRNAs are small stretches of RNA that can bind an inhibit expression of target genes. As such, miR-210 is used as a biomarker for tumor hypoxia and is generally correlated with a worse prognosis. miRNAs bind mRNA to block their transcription, and miR-201 binds mRNAs that are needed for mitochondrial activity. miR-210 can also stabilize HIF-1α, which allows the transcription factor to bind and activate hypoxia-inducing genes. In this way, miR-210 can also contribute to increase hypoxia [46].

7. Conclusion

Obesity can contribute to cancer progression through a variety of mechanisms. However, the main effects of obesity in the context of cancer are activation of pathways that lead to drug resistance, inflammation, and dysregulation of sex hormones and adipokines. The adipokine leptin plays a central role in the contribution of obesity to cancer progression, as it is over-expressed in obesity and contributes to insulin secretion and inflammation. Estrogen, IGF-1, and inflammatory factors also play pivotal roles cancer progression in the context obesity. However, the mechanisms discussed in this chapter are by no means an exhaustive list of what is known, and more research must still be done to completely understand the interplay between adipose tissue and the tumor microenvironment.

Author details

Nicole Bonan and Katie DeCicco-Skinner*
Department of Biology, American University, Washington, DC, United States

*Address all correspondence to: decicco@american.edu

References

[1] Centers for Disease Control and Prevention. Adult Obesity Facts [Internet]. 2017. Available from: https://www.cdc.gov/obesity/data/adult.html [Accessed: Jun 8, 2018]

[2] World Health Organization. Obesity and Overweight Fact Sheet [Internet]. 2018. Available from: http://www.who.int/news-room/fact-sheets/detail/obesity-and-overweight [Accessed: Jul 13, 2018]

[3] Garg SK, Maurer H, Reed K, Selagamsetty R. Diabetes and cancer: Two diseases with obesity as a common risk factor. Diabetes, Obesity, and Metabolism. 2014;**16**:97-110. DOI: 10.1111/dom.12124

[4] Basen-Engquist K, Chang M. Obesity and cancer risk: Recent review and evidence. Current Oncology Reports. 2011;**13**:71-76. DOI: 10.1007/s11912-010-0139-7

[5] De Pergola G, Silvestris F. Obesity as a major risk factor for cancer. Journal of Obesity. 2013;**2013**:1-11. DOI: 10.1155/2013/291546

[6] Ligibel JA, Alfano CM, Courneya KS, Demark-Wahnefried W, Burger RA, et al. American Society of Clinical Oncology statement on obesity and cancer. Journal of Clinical Oncology. 2014;**32**:3568-3574. DOI: 10.1200/JCO.2014.58.4680

[7] O'Flanagan CH, Bowers LW, Hursting SD. A weighty problem: Metabolic perturbations and the obesity-cancer link. Hormone Molecular Biology and Clinical Investigation. 2016;**23**:47-57. DOI: 10.1515/hmbci-2015-0022

[8] Park J, Morley TS, Kim M, Clegg DJ, Scherer PE. Obesity and cancer—Mechanisms underlying tumor progression and recurrence. Nature Reviews Endocrinology. 2015;**10**: 455-465. DOI: 10.1038/nrendo.2014.94

[9] Onstad MA, Schmandt RE, Lu KH. Addressing the role of obesity in endometrial cancer risk, prevention, and treatment. Journal of Clinical Oncology. 2016;**34**:4225-4230. DOI: 10.1200/JCO.2016.69.4638

[10] Aleksandrova K, Stelmach-Mardas M, Schlesinger S. Obesity and liver cancer. Recent Results in Cancer Research. 2014;**10**:455-465. DOI: 10.1038/nrendo.2014.94

[11] Preziosi G, Oben JA, Fusai G. Obesity and pancreatic cancer. Surgical Oncology. 2014;**23**:61-71. DOI: 10.1016/j.suronc.2014.02.003

[12] Bardou M, Barkun AN, Martel M. Obesity and colorectal cancer. Gut. 2013;**62**:933-947. DOI: 10.1136/gutjnl-2013-304701

[13] Vidal AC, Howard LE, Moreira DM, Castro-Santamaria R, Andriole GL Jr, Freedland SJ. Obesity increases the risk for high-grade prostate cancer: Results from the REDUCE study. Cancer Epidemiology, Biomarkers and Prevention. 2014;**23**:2936-2942. DOI: 10.1158/1055-9965.EPI-1
4-0795

[14] Chan DC, Norat T. Obesity and breast cancer: Not only a risk factor. Current Treatment Options in Oncology. 2015;**16**:22. DOI: 10.1007/s11864-015-0341-9

[15] Bullwinkle EM, Parker MD, Bonan NF, Falkenberg LG, Davison SP, DeCicco-Skinner KL. Adipocytes contribute to the growth and progression of multiple myeloma: Unraveling obesity related differences in adipocyte signaling. Cancer Letters. 2016;**380**:114-121. DOI: 10.1016/j.canlet.2016.06.101

[16] National Cancer Institute at the National Institutes of Health. Cancers Associated with Overweight and Obesity [Internet]. Available from: https://www.cancer.gov/about-cancer/causes-prevention/risk/obesity/overweight-cancers-infographic [Accessed: Jun 8, 2018]

[17] Deng T, Lyon CJ, Bergin S, Caligiuri MA, Hsueh WA. Obesity, inflammation, and cancer. Annual Review of Pathology: Mechanisms of Disease. 2016;**11**:421-449. DOI: 10.1146/annurev-pathol-012615-044359

[18] Shuster A, Patlas M, Pinthus JH, Mourtzakis M. The clinical importance of visceral adiposity: A clinical review of methods for visceral adipose tissue analysis. The British Journal of Radiology. 2012;**85**:1-10. DOI: 10.1259/bjr/38447238

[19] Ibrahim MM. Subutaneous and visceral adipose tissue: Structural and functional differences. Obesity Reviews. 2010;**11**:11-18. DOI: 10.1111/j.1467-789X.2009.00623.x

[20] Zhang C, Rexrode KM, van Dam RM, Li TY, Hu FB. Abdominal obesity and the risk of all-cause, cardiovascular, and cancer mortality: Sixteen years of follow-up in US women. Circulation. 2008;**117**:1656-1667. DOI: 10.1161/CIRCULATIONHA.107.739714

[21] Ebadi M, Martin L, Ghosh S, Field CJ, Lehner R, Baracos VE, Mazurak VC. Subcutaneous adiposity is an independent predictor of mortality in cancer patients. British Journal of Cancer. 2017;**117**:148-155. DOI: 10.1038/bjc.2017.149

[22] De Meyts P. The insulin receptor and its signal transduction network. In: De Groot LJ, Chrousos G, Dungan K, et al., editors. Endotext. South Dartmouth: MDText.com, Inc.; 2016

[23] Malaguarnera R, Belfiore A. The insulin receptor: A new target for cancer therapy. Frontiers in Endocrinology. 2011;**2**:93. DOI: 10.3389/fendo.2011.00093

[24] Hopkins BD, Goncalves MD, Cantley LC. Obesity and cancer mechanisms: Cancer metabolism. Journal of Clinical Oncology. 2016;**34**:4277-4283. DOI: 10.1200/JCO.2016.67.9712

[25] Haeusler RA, McGraw TE, Accili D. Biochemical and cellular properties of insulin receptor signaling. Nature Reviews. 2017;**19**:31-44. DOI: 10.1038/nrm.2017.89

[26] Tarasiuk A, Mosinska P, Fichna J. The mechanisms linking obesity to colon cancer: An overview. Obesity Research and Clinical Practice. 2018. DOI: 10.1016/j.orcp.2018.01.005

[27] Allard JB, Duan C. IGF-binding proteins: Why do they exist and why are there so many? Frontiers in Endocrinology. 2018;**9**:1-12. DOI: 10.3389/ fendo.2018.00117

[28] King H, Aleksic T, Haluska P, Macaulay VM. Can we unlock the potential of IGF-1R inhibition in cancer therapy? Cancer Treatment Reviews. 2014;**40**:1096-1105. DOI: 10.1016/j.ctrv.2014.07.004

[29] Davaadelger B, Duna L, Perez R, Gitelis S, Maki CG. Crosstalk between the IFD-1R/AKT/mTORC1 pathway and the tumor suppressors p53 and p27 determines cisplatin sensitivity and limits the effectiveness of an IGF-1R pathway inhibitor. Oncotarget. 2016;**7**:27511-27526. DOI: 10.18632/oncotarget.8484

[30] Pernicova I, Korbonits M. Metformin—Mode of action and clinical implications for diabetes and cancer. Nature Reviews Endocrinology. 2014;**10**:143-156. DOI: 10.1038/nrendo.2013.256

[31] Schulster M, Bernie AM, Ramasamy R. The role of estradiol in male reproductive function. Asian Journal of Andrology. 2016;**18**:435-440. DOI: 10.4103/1008-682X.173932

[32] Tubbs A, Nussenzweig A. Endogenous DNA damage as a source of genomic instability in cancer. Cell. 2017;**168**:644-656. DOI: 10.1016/j.cell.2017.01.002

[33] Lumachi F, Brunello A, Maruzzo A, Basso U, Basso SM. Treatment of estrogen receptor-positive breast cancer. Current Medicinal Chemistry. 2013;**20**:596-604. DOI: 10.2174/092986713804999303

[34] Picon-Ruiz M, Morata-Tarifa C, Valle-Goffin JJ, Friedman ER, Slingerland JM. Obesity and adverse breast cancer risk and outcome: Mechanistic insights and strategies for intervention. CA: A Cancer Journal for Clinicians. 2017;**67**:378-397. DOI: 10.3322/caac.21405

[35] Stork CT, Bocek M, Crossley MP, Sollier J, Sanz LA, Chedin F, Swigut T, Cimprich KA. Co-transcriptional R-loops are the main cause of estrogen-induced DNA damage. eLIFE Sciences. 2016;**5**:1-21. e17548. DOI: 10.7554/eLife.17548

[36] Newman G, Gonzalez-Perez RR. Leptin-cytokine crosstalk in breast cancer. Molecular and Cellular Endocrinology. 2014;**382**:570-582. DOI: 10.1016/j.mce.2013.03.025

[37] Dalamaga M, Diakopoulos KN, Mantzoros CS. The role of adiponectin in cancer: A review of current evidence. Endocrine Reviews. 2012;**33**:547-594. DOI: 10.1210/er.2011-1015

[38] DeCicco-Skinner KL, Nolan SJ, Deshpande MM, Trovato EL, Dempsey TA, Wiest JS. Altered prostanoid signaling contributes to increased skin tumorigenesis in Tpl2 knockout mice. PLoS One. 2013;**8**:e56212. DOI: 10.1371/journal.pone.0056212

[39] Abbas AK, Lichtman AH, Pillai S. Differentiation and functions of CD4+ effector T cells. In: Cellular and Molecular Immunology. 8th ed. Philadelphia: Elsevier Saunders; 2015. pp. 213-230

[40] Gerriets VA, MacIver NJ. Role of T cells in malnutrition and obesity. Frontiers in Immunoloy. 2014;**5**:379. DOI: 10.3389/fimmu.2014.00379

[41] Corrêa LH, Corrêa R, Farinasso CM, de Sant'Ana Dourado LP, Magalhães KG. Adipocytes and macrophages interplay in the orchestration of tumor microenvironment: New implications in cancer research. Frontiers in Immunology. 2017;**8**:1129. DOI: 10.3389/fimmu.201701129

[42] Kouidhi S, Noman MZ, Kieda C, Elgaaied AB, Chouaib S. Intrinsic and tumor microenvironment-induced metabolism adaptations of T cells and impact on their differentiation and function. Frontiers in Immunology. 2016;**7**:114. DOI: 10.3389/fummu.2016.00114

[43] Pucino V, De Rosa V, Procaccini C, Matarese G. Regulatory T cells, leptin, and angiogenesis. In: Marone G, Granat F, editors. Angiogenesis, Lymphangiogenesis and Clinical Implications. Basel: Karger; 2016. pp. 155-169. DOI: 10.1159/000353557

[44] Ladoire S, Martin F, Ghiringhelli F. Prognostic role of FOXP3+ regulatory T cells infiltrating human carcinomas: The paradox of colorectal cancer. Cancer Immunology, Immunotherapy. 2011;**60**:909-918. DOI: 10.1007/s00262-011-1046-y

[45] Rothenberger NJ, Somasundaram A, Stabile LP. The role of the estrogen

pathway in the tumor microenvironment. International Journal of Molecular Sciences. 2018;**19**: 1-16. DOI: 10.3390/ijms19020611

[46] Diedrich J, Gusky HC, Podgorski I. Adipose tissue dysfunction and its effects on tumor metabolism. Hormone Molecular Biology and Clinical Investigation. 2015;**21**:17-41. DOI: 10.1515/hmbci-2014-0045

Chapter 4

Reproductive Consequences of Obesity

Tamara Hunter and Roger Hart

Abstract

With increasing global obesity, there is a growing body of research looking at the impact of this on reproduction. Both male and female fertility are impacted on by being overweight or obese. Although the pathophysiology is not clear, it appears that obesity impacts endocrine function in men and women, oocyte and sperm quality, embryo quality, endocrine receptivity, and implantation. Miscarriage, pregnancy, and live birth rates and the risk of congenital malformations are all influenced by obesity. Transgenerational health is also affected, with metabolic, endocrine, and reproductive outcomes in the offspring being negatively affected by both paternal and maternal obesity. It appears that weight loss results in improvements in these outcomes and various strategies have been employed including lifestyle and behavior modification, pharmacological agents, and also bariatric surgery. This chapter aims to explore the reproductive outcomes of obesity and how this can be best managed to improve outcomes.

Keywords: obesity, IVF, embryos, bariatric, fertility, offspring, reproduction, lifestyle, oocyte, sperm

1. Introduction

Overweight or obesity is defined as an accumulation of excess body fat that poses a risk for health [1]. A measure often used in assessment of this is the body mass index (BMI), which is a person's weight in kilograms divided by height in meters squared (kg/m^2). Obesity is a BMI greater than 30 and overweight is a BMI greater than 25, although in South East Asian populations, it is generally accepted that the upper limit of normal is a BMI of 23.

Globally, 39% of adults over 18 years are overweight and 13% are obese, and worldwide, obesity has tripled since the 1970s [2]. Being overweight or obese is directly linked to a greater risk of mortality and disease than being underweight.

Infertility is defined as failure to achieve a clinical pregnancy after 12 months or more of regular unprotected sexual intercourse [3]. Globally, at least 50 million couples worldwide experience infertility, with the burden affecting up to one in four couples in developing nations. The overall prevalence of infertility does not appear to have changed since the 1990s.

Overweight or obesity is understood to impact on both female and male reproductive health, and mounting research demonstrates that this impact will extend to the health and reproductive outcomes of future generations.

 IntechOpen

2. Effects of obesity on female reproduction

2.1 Hormonal effects of obesity

Menstrual irregularities occur more frequently in women who are overweight. This is due to a functional alteration to the hypothalamic-pituitary-ovarian (HPO) axis from various factors. Firstly, obesity induces a hyperinsulinemic state, separate to polycystic ovarian syndrome (PCOS). Hyperinsulinemia leads to a suppression in serum hormone binding globulin (SHBG), which results in an increase in bioactive androgens. These androgens are subsequently aromatized within body fat to estrogen, which suppresses gonadotrophins produced by the pituitary [4].

Elevated androgens in PCOS also lead to an increased deposition of visceral fat, exacerbating insulin resistance and hyperinsulinemia, further stimulating androgen production and perpetuating the cycle of pituitary suppression [5].

Additionally, adipokines, cytokines produced from adipose tissue, are known to impact on ovulation. Obese women have higher levels of circulating leptin, a cell-signaling protein from adipose tissue, than normal weight women, and this can therefore mean a chronic downregulation of the receptor in the hypothalamus, [6] resulting in suppression of the HPO axis activity. A study of eumenorrheic obese women demonstrated that the amplitude of luteinizing hormone (LH) pulses was significantly reduced compared with normal weight women, again pointing to a central defect [7].

Obese women remain subfertile even if they are ovulatory. Two studies in large cohorts of Danish women showed a decline in fecundability ratios with increasing BMI [8, 9]. Another large American cohort [10] along with a Dutch cohort of over 3000 women [11] also demonstrated a linear decline in spontaneous conception rates with rising BMI.

Consequently, there are other factors at play that affect fertility in overweight and obese women.

2.2 Effects of obesity on oocyte quality

Data show that being overweight or obese can have profound impact on oocyte quality. A study of over 45,000 assisted reproduction transfers demonstrated that a higher BMI resulted in a lower likelihood of successful pregnancy when autologous oocytes were used but not when oocytes from lean donors were used [12]. This has been demonstrated in other research as well [13].

Studies also suggest that obese women in in vitro fertilization (IVF) cycles require higher levels of gonadotrophin stimulation and longer treatment to achieve an oocyte retrieval [14]. This is also the case in superovulation for intrauterine insemination cycles [15]. Obese women also have a greater risk of cycle cancelation, lesser oocytes collected, and lesser oocyte maturity than normal weight women [16–18].

Several mechanisms are believed to impact on the oocyte quality in obese women.

Obesity is an inflammatory state where women have higher circulating levels of C-reactive protein (CRP), which is an inflammatory biomarker. Adipose tissue produces many proinflammatory adipokines including leptin, tumor necrosis factor alpha (TNFα), and interleukin (IL) 6. The reproductive tissues, like all tissues, are negatively affected by inflammation. The follicular environment is altered in an obese woman. Follicular fluid contains higher levels of insulin, triglycerides, leptin, and markers of inflammation such as lactate and CRP [6]. Leptin affects steroidogenic pathways in granulosa cells, thus affecting estrogen and progesterone production. This could therefore have impact downstream on endometrial receptivity and implantation [6].

In obese mouse models, the ovaries demonstrate more apoptotic follicles and the oocytes themselves are smaller and less likely to be mature. These oocytes reveal high rates of meiotic aneuploidy due to fragmented and disorganized meiotic spindles and chromosomes that are not properly aligned on the metaphase plate [6].

Independent from this, obesity alters mitochondrial function in the oocyte. In an obese mouse model, the mitochondria have a disordered architecture with fewer cristae, more vacuoles, and evidence of swelling [19]. These abnormal mitochondria show evidence of metabolic stress, which leads to a compensatory increase in mitochondrial DNA copy number in obese mice [6, 20]. Obese mice also demonstrate evidence of endoplasmic reticulum (ER) stress where their cumulous-oocyte complexes have increased ER stress markers and increased granulosa cell apoptosis [21].

A possible cause for this cellular and organelle damage in obesity is lipotoxicity. Lipotoxicity is a condition where fatty acids from the diet that exceed the storage ability of the adipocytes can accumulate in other tissues and cause toxic effects.

Obese women have higher circulating free fatty acids (FFAs), which increase reactive oxygen species (ROS) that induce mitochondrial and ER stress and leads to apoptosis. Studies have shown that the oocytes of mice have significant increased production of ROS along with depleted glutathione levels, which is an important intracellular antioxidant defense against ROS [22]. Oocytes exposed to maternal obesity or to high levels of FFA in vitro have demonstrated perturbed mitochondria with reduced mitochondrial function, which then fail to support normal cleavage and embryo development [21].

2.3 Effects of obesity on embryo quality

The preimplantation embryo is also affected by an obese environment. Given that the early embryonic development is largely driven by the oocyte, it is not unexpected that if the oocyte is negatively affected, then the embryo development would be too.

In a mouse model, embryos of obese females have demonstrated slower preimplantation development and disordered differentiation to inner cell mass and trophectoderm lineage [20].

In an IVF model with autologous oocytes, obese women are more likely to create poor quality embryos [23, 24]. One study noted that embryos from women with a BMI > 25 kg/m^2 were less likely to develop after fertilization and those that did reached the morula stage more rapidly. Those that reached the blastocyst stage had fewer cells in the trophectoderm and demonstrated poor glucose uptake and increased levels of triglycerides along with altered amino acid metabolism compared with embryos from normal weight women (BMI < 25 kg/m^2) [25].

Much like oocytes, embryos may also be susceptible to lipotoxicity. Murine embryos that are cultured in palmitic acid, the most common FFA present in human serum, have fewer nuclei and altered IGF-1 receptor expression [26]. This negatively affects insulin sensitivity and glucose transport at a critical stage in development. This study also demonstrated that the trophoblastic cells that are exposed to the palmitic acid proliferate less and undergo apoptosis in a dose-dependent fashion.

Elevated leptin levels also have a direct negative effect on the developing embryo. In vitro studies have demonstrated that leptin has a stimulating effect on human trophoblastic cell growth and inhibition of leptin decreases that proliferation and induces apoptosis [27]. Much like its effect in the brain, tonically elevated leptin levels in an obese state may decrease the sensitivity of trophoblastic cells to its effect, altering their development.

However, there are studies in human models that have not demonstrated a negative effect of obesity on embryo quality, showing no significant difference in the quality of transferred embryos between the different BMI groups [28–31]. Although it is worth noting that despite the quality of transferred embryos being similar, other studies have suggested a reduction in the overall quality of all embryos created in an IVF cycle [14, 24], with fewer surplus embryos cryopreserved in an obese population compared to women with a normal BMI [14]. A retrospective analysis of IVF/ICSI cycles observed that in young women, obesity led to a significant reduction in average embryo quality, cryopreservation, and also embryo utilization [24]. A large retrospective analysis of over 6500 IVF cycles demonstrated no difference in embryo quality but did comment that there were poorer outcomes in the obese women [31]. Certainly, large prospective trials are required to further elucidate the effect of obesity on the embryo.

2.4 Effects of obesity on endometrial receptivity and implantation

There are conflicting data as to whether or not obesity affects endometrial receptivity and implantation of embryos, and there are several suggested mechanisms.

Leukemia inhibitory factor (LIF) has been implicated in the regulation of implantation, and a significant negative correlation between endometrial glandular LIF and BMI has been observed [32]. It has also been suggested that a state of relative hyperestrogenemia that is seen in obese women (due to aromatization of androgens to estrogen in adipose tissue) may also have a detrimental effect on receptivity [32].

Obesity is associated with insulin resistance and hyperinsulinemia. Elevated insulin levels have been associated with a reduction on glycodelin and insulin-like growth factor binding protein 1 (IGFBP1). Low levels of glycodelin have been associated with recurrent pregnancy loss, and IGFBP1 is an integral molecule involved in adhesion during implantation [32]. Derangement in these molecules may contribute to reduced receptivity in obese women.

As noted previously, obesity is an inflammatory state and obese women have been observed to have elevations in proinflammatory cytokines (IL6, TNFα), and these inflammatory markers are thought to exert negative effects on implantation [14].

Obese women also have a different pattern of endometrial gene expression during implantation than lean women [33], which is more pronounced when examined in the context of infertility. It is postulated that this is due to all or some of the abovementioned factors and the change in the intrauterine milieu of the obese women.

Although there are several plausible mechanisms as to how obesity impacts negatively on endometrial receptivity and implantation, the data for impact on infertility are inconsistent and contradictory. The best model for discriminating between the obesity effects on oocyte/embryo and endometrium is the oocyte donation model [34]. A retrospective review of over 2500 oocyte donation cycles demonstrated a negative trend in pregnancy rates with a rising BMI and a statistically significantly lower pregnancy rate in overweight and obese women compared to normal weight women [35]. However, the implantation rates were considered similar, suggesting the difference between groups was due to an increased pregnancy loss rate in the obese women. Another study also demonstrated lower live birth rates among obese surrogates compared to normal weight women [36]. Other smaller studies have suggested no difference in outcomes in obese oocyte recipients [37].

A case-controlled trial looking at IVF with autologous oocytes observed that women with a BMI > 25 kg/m^2 had reduced implantation and pregnancy rates along with increased miscarriage rates [38]. Once again, large well-designed prospective studies using this model are required to further examine the effect of obesity on endometrial receptivity and implantation.

2.5 Effects of obesity on miscarriage

The role of obesity and miscarriage is also debated. Given the recognized impact of obesity on both the embryo and the endometrium, it is a reasonable assumption that miscarriage rates would be higher in an overweight and obese population.

Several studies have demonstrated ever-increasing odds of miscarriage with increasing BMI, in ovulation induction for anovulatory infertility, as well as in IVF cycles in both fresh and frozen cycles [28, 17, 39, 40]. A large meta-analysis of over 47,000 cycles confirmed that overweight or obese women have a higher rate of miscarriage compared with normal weight women [41]. This has also been demonstrated in donor oocyte cycles, with higher miscarriage rates in obese recipients than in normal weight women [42].

Interestingly, however, a larger follow-up study of over 2600 donor oocyte cycles by the same group [43] did not demonstrate a difference in miscarriage rates. There was a trend toward a negative impact; however, it was only when a composite measure of ongoing pregnancy rate per cycle was calculated that this was shown to be significantly lower in the obese population.

A meta-analysis looking at both spontaneous and assisted reproduction pregnancies showed that women with a BMI > 25 kg/m^2 had a significantly higher rate of miscarriage <20 weeks gestation. Subgroup analysis confirmed this to be in the donor oocyte cycles but not across all patients in the studies [44]. Another study demonstrated that in a group of women with a history of recurrent pregnancy loss (RPL), obesity is a well-recognized risk factor for miscarriage in a subsequent pregnancy [45].

A striking study looking at the chromosomal make-up of miscarried specimens from patients with RPL demonstrated that obese women had a much higher rate of euploid pregnancy loss compared to normal weight women. This supports the theory of the impact of obesity on embryo quality and endometrial receptivity.

3. Effects of obesity on male reproduction

Historically, the impact of obesity on reproduction has largely been researched in female populations with very little examination of the impact of male obesity. There is, however, a growing body of research to indicate that obesity in the male is a cause for concern. A systematic review of 30 studies with over 115,000 participants found that obese men were more likely to experience infertility and that clinical pregnancy and live birth rates per assisted reproduction cycle were reduced.

3.1 Hormonal effects of male obesity

Much like in the female, the hypothalamic-pituitary-gonadal (HPG) axis is dysregulated in the setting of male obesity. There is strong evidence of a negative effect of obesity on total testosterone, SHBG, and free testosterone [46] as well as reduced inhibin B concentrations and diminished luteinizing hormone (LH) pulse amplitude [4]. It is well understood that suppression of SHBG by hyperinsulinemia in obese men increases androgen availability for aromatization to estrogen in adipose tissue, which may then lead to negative feedback and reduction in gonadotrophin secretion [4]. Consequent to this is a decreased Leydig cell testosterone secretion, which ultimately affects spermatogenesis.

The function of the Sertoli cell, which provides both physical and nutritional support to the developing germ cell, is also impacted. Adhesion of the Sertoli cell is dependent on testosterone, and a reduction in these levels can lead to retention and phagocytosis of mature spermatids and ultimately reduced sperm counts. Other hormones that influence Sertoli cell function, FSH, LH, inhibin B, and SHBG are all lower in obese men [47].

3.2 Effects of obesity on spermatogenesis

The best markers to assess the impact of obesity on spermatogenesis are the sperm parameters from the semen analysis (count, motility, and morphology). Rodent models clearly demonstrate that diet-induced male obesity leads to reduced sperm motility, decreased sperm count, and decreased percentage of sperm with normal morphology [47], though some argue that this is indirectly due to altered hormonal stimulation.

The impact of male obesity on sperm parameters in humans is more controversial, with many contradicting studies. A review of studies [47] demonstrated varying results for the impact of male obesity on sperm concentration, morphology, and motility. The reviewers commented that there were several significant confounders including lifestyle factors such as smoking and alcohol consumption as well as cofactors such as the metabolic syndrome, which have all been shown to impact on sperm parameters. Most of the cohorts studied come from fertility centers and so are biased toward subfertile men, who may differ from the background population. Additionally, many studies rely on self-reporting, which can lead to inaccuracies.

A recent systematic review that evaluated 21 studies demonstrated a J-shaped correlation between male obesity and sperm count, whereby overweight and obesity is associated with higher rates of oligozoospermia and azoospermia [48].

3.3 Effects of obesity on sperm DNA integrity

In addition to sperm parameters, sperm DNA integrity has been found to be an important factor for the ability of a sperm to generate a healthy pregnancy [49]. Reactive oxygen species (ROS), commonly elevated in subfertile men, have been found to impair sperm DNA integrity. This is likely due to the fact that sperm are highly susceptible to ROS in the later stages of spermiogenesis as they lose the majority of their antioxidant defenses when they shed cytoplasm (**Figure 1**).

Studies have demonstrated that there is a positive correlation between increasing adiposity and higher sperm and seminal plasma ROS levels [50–52]. Oxidative stress is highly correlated with cumulative damage in the body induced by free radicals that are inadequately neutralized by antioxidant mechanisms. Antioxidant enzymes include superoxide dismutase (SOD), catalase (CAT), and glutathione S-transferase (GST). A recent study in an obese mouse model showed decreased SOD in the testicular tissues of obese rats [53].

Studies have also confirmed that male obesity is associated with higher levels of sperm DNA damage [47], due to the oxygen-free radical damage, and a direct thermal effect on the testicles due to obesity. It is therefore a reasonable assumption that male obesity negatively impacts on sperm DNA integrity via high ROS levels within the testis. DNA fragmentation has been proven to reduce male fertility, possibly reduce success with assisted reproduction, and increase pregnancy loss.

Although not directly impacting on testicular function, obesity leading to reduced testosterone results in a reduction in libido and negatively impacts on erectile and ejaculatory function, which all lead to a reduction in fecundity [54].

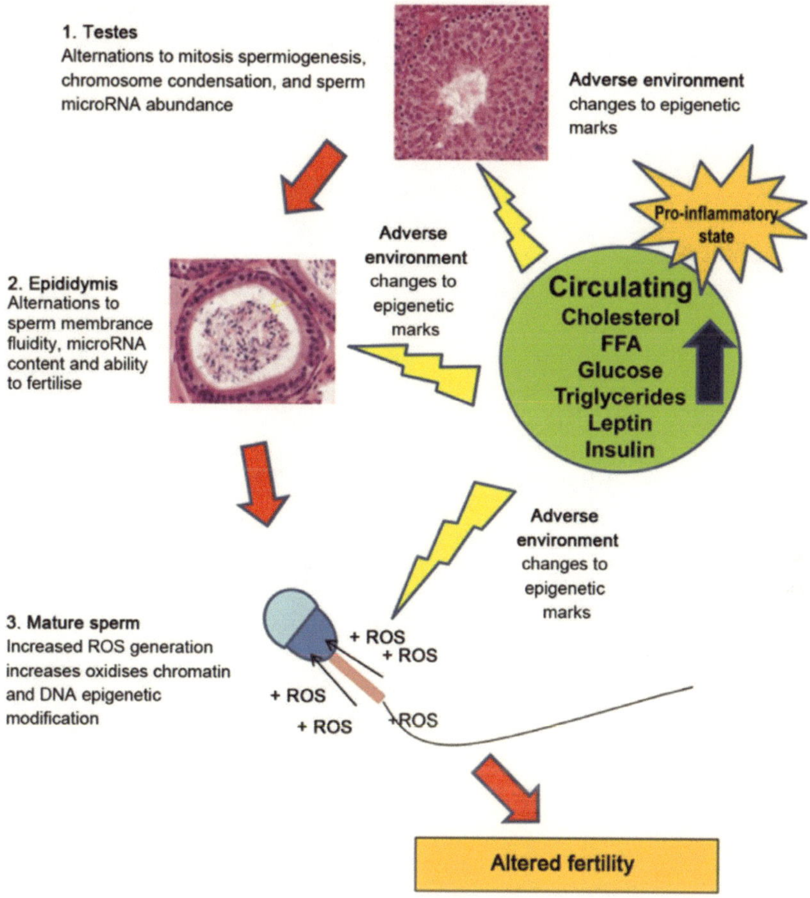

Figure 1.
Hypothesis on how epigenetic changes and impact of ROS due to an obese proinflammatory environment can occur at multiple different points along the development of the sperm, resulting in altered fertility [47].

4. Transgenerational effects of parental obesity

There is good evidence to show that maternal obesity during pregnancy is a risk factor for obesity in the offspring [55]. There is also an increasing body of evidence that obesity in males and females periconceptionally can impact on the metabolic health and even fertility of future generations. By using animal models, the impact of maternal and paternal obesity on offspring and future generations has been examined. Studies have demonstrated that obesity and other health conditions can be transmitted across multiple generations via epigenetic mechanisms down either the maternal or the paternal line.

An elegant murine study by Huypens and others [56] induced obesity in both male and female parents for 6 weeks with a high-fat diet (HFD) and then performed IVF. Embryos created from all combinations of parents were transferred into a lean dam, to negate the impact of obesity during pregnancy (**Figure 2**).

Female offspring born from both maternal and paternal obese parents gained more weight than the male offspring. The risk of female offspring obesity was reduced if only the female parent was obese, suggesting an additive effect.

Females from obese parents also had significant metabolic derangements. They demonstrated a delay in blood glucose clearance leading to hyperinsulinemia and increased fat mass. Male offspring demonstrated severe insulin resistance before

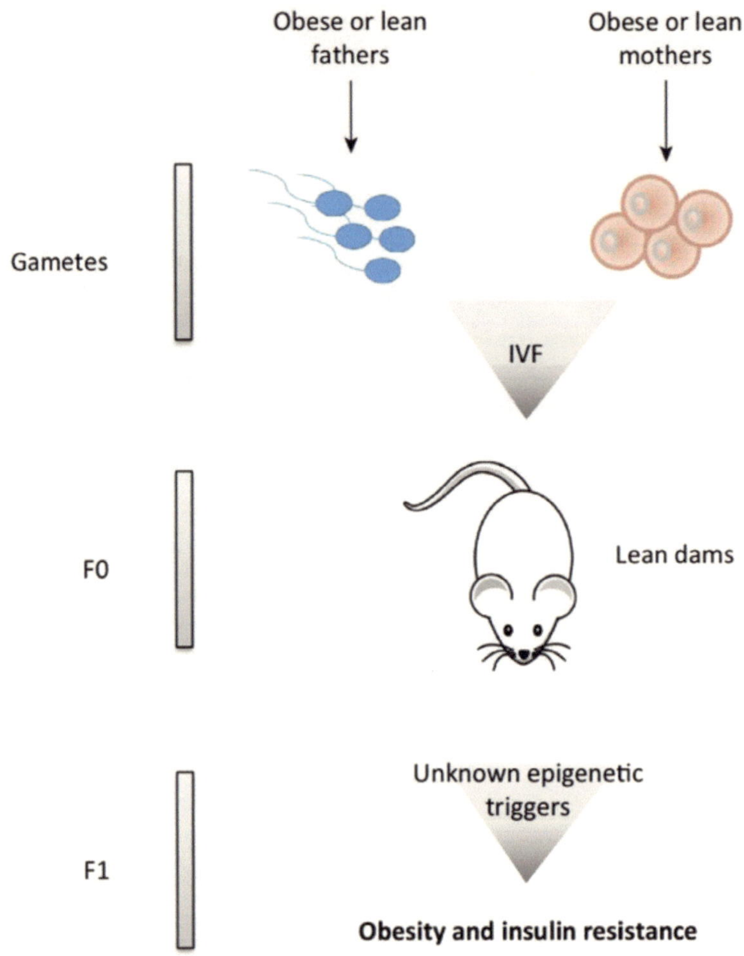

Figure 2.
Embryos created from different combinations of obese and lean parents were transferred into a lean surrogate dam, to determine the impact of overweight and obesity in male and female parents on the next generation [55].

any change in body weight. This insulin resistance was acquired in the offspring via the maternal line.

Another study by Fullston and others [57] demonstrated that paternal obesity initiated changes to metabolic health and obesity in multiple subsequent generations. Insulin resistance and obesity were transmitted to both the female and male first-generation offspring and then through both parental lineages to the second generation with amplified obesity in the female offspring in the first generation and in their sons in the second generation.

Epigenetics is the hypothesized mechanism for transgenerational disease patterns. It was thought that this was in utero exposure to epigenetic modification of offspring DNA or histone modification during developmental stages without alteration to the DNA itself. However, this has been broadened to include transgenerational (meiotic) alterations and occurs through several possible processes including DNA methylation, histone modification, DNA-binding proteins, and noncoding RNA [6] (**Figure 1**).

In the study by Fullston and others [57], they demonstrated that diet-induced paternal obesity leads to an alteration in mRNAs and microRNAs within the rodent testes, with alteration in the sperm microRNA content as well. They also detected

25% reduction in global methylation of germ cell DNA. These modifications are potential signals to program obesity and impaired metabolic health in offspring. These effects have also been demonstrated in humans with hypomethylation of sperm being associated with subfertility [58]. Another study [59] demonstrated, in a mouse model of diet-induced obesity, sperm tRNA-derived small RNAs impaired offspring glucose tolerance and induced insulin resistance. Other studies have also demonstrated that both maternal and paternal obesity can cause epigenetic changes that predispose offspring to obesity or metabolic disease later in life [60].

5. Effectiveness of weight loss strategies

There is no doubt that obesity contributes to significant periconceptional and perinatal morbidity and has been clearly associated with prolonged time to conception, increased pregnancy loss, and higher rates of adverse pregnancy outcomes such as preeclampsia and gestational diabetes along with preterm birth and in turn increased fetal morbidity and mortality. As mentioned previously, there is increasing information that it affects fertility and miscarriage rates so it is not unexpected that national and international guidelines focus on weight loss prior to either spontaneous conception or assisted reproduction [4, 32, 61] and that first-line management is ideally with lifestyle intervention and behavior modification.

5.1 Lifestyle intervention and behavior modification

It is controversial as to whether weight loss through dietary intervention, exercise programs, or behavior modification will impact significantly on spontaneous conception rates or success with assisted reproduction. There are a group of studies that suggest improved ovulatory frequency, pregnancy rates, and cost per pregnancy achieved in assisted reproduction [32, 62]. One randomized controlled trial demonstrated that a 12-week diet and exercise program resulted in a mean weight loss of 5.4 kg in the intervention group, a trend toward a higher clinical pregnancy rate and a significant difference in live birth rates [63]. A secondary analysis of two parallel randomized controlled trials in obese PCOS women also demonstrated that deferred ovulation induction treatment preceded by lifestyle modification resulted in significantly improved ovulation rates and live birth rates when compared with immediate treatment [62]. Weight reduction in an obese anovulatory population has been shown to improve pregnancy rates. A 6-month lifestyle intervention induced an average weight loss of 10 kg, which resulted in return of ovulation in 90% of participants and 78% conceiving. The miscarriage rate was 18% [64].

However, other studies suggest surprisingly little impact on conception and fertility outcomes. One large multicenter randomized controlled trial involving a 12-week intensive dietary intervention followed by IVF demonstrated a significant weight reduction in the intervention group, but this was not reflected in reproductive outcomes [65]. Live birth rates through IVF and miscarriage rates were not significantly different. The authors did note that the spontaneous pregnancy rates in the intervention group compared to the immediate treatment group were significantly higher. This may, however, have been due to having a longer time to achieve a spontaneous pregnancy, albeit they were then older at the time of IVF [65].

Firstly, lifestyle modification often results in only a modest weight loss. In a general population large-scale disease prevention programs including intensive counseling, support, and changes in diet and exercise, a 4–6 kg weight loss could be achieved but was sufficient to reduce the incidence of diabetes and metabolic syndrome [66]. Unfortunately, achieved weight loss is often regained relatively quickly [61]. It is reported that weight loss through behavior modification and lifestyle change of greater than 10% and sustained for longer than 12 months occurs in only 20% of individuals who start a program [67].

Additionally, lifestyle modification has been attributed to positive effects on the endocrine and metabolic profile of an individual and that this, and not the weight loss, is the cause of the reported improved reproductive outcomes [68]. As such, there is a call for caution on delaying fertility treatment to allow lifestyle modification and weight loss to occur [69].

5.2 Pharmacological agents

Due to the modest weight loss from lifestyle intervention, pharmacotherapy is required as an adjunct to deliver better outcomes. There is good evidence to show that it can be used to help manage hypertension, diabetes, and cardiovascular disease in the obese population when used in addition to not replacing lifestyle intervention.

National and international bodies concur that these pharmacological agents can be used to help with weight loss prior to conceiving in those who are obese or those who are overweight with associated weight-related coexisting conditions [4, 32, 61]. It is important to note, however, that none of these drugs have been studied in men or women before conception and their effects on menstrual cycles, ovulation, or even pregnancy rates are unknown.

Phentermine is a sympathomimetic agent that suppresses appetite. Studies have indicated significant weight loss at 6 months compared to placebo [70]. There are side effects of dry mouth, agitation, insomnia, and tachycardia, and it is not recommended in patients with a history of cardiovascular disease. It is the most commonly used weight loss drug in Australia and the USA.

Orlistat inhibits pancreatic and gastric lipases and so reduces the absorption of dietary fats. It is found to be effective for weight loss [71] but has the side effects of fat malabsorption including steatorrhea, fecal incontinence, and fat-soluble vitamin deficiency [72].

Liraglutide is a glucagon-like peptide-1 agonist and controls hyperglycemia without causing hypoglycemia or weight gain. This drug was initially used to treat type 2 diabetes mellitus but its side effect profile of decreased appetite and subsequent weight loss led to its use as a weight loss agent. Studies demonstrate significant weight loss over placebo and improvement on cardiometabolic parameters [73]. Common side effects are nausea, vomiting, and diarrhea, which are dose related and diminish over time.

Topiramate, an anticonvulsant, has also been used to treat obesity due to the side effect of weight loss and is used as either monotherapy or in combination with phentermine. A naltrexone/bupropion combination has also been demonstrated to provide average weight loss over 12 months [74], and Lorcaserin, a selective 5-hydroxytryptamine 2c receptor agonist, also suppresses appetite with a 3.6% weight loss over a year [75].

All of these agents are contraindicated in pregnancy.

One agent not contraindicated in pregnancy is metformin. Metformin is a biguanide that inhibits hepatic glucose production and increases peripheral tissue sensitivity to insulin, resulting in a reduced circulating insulin and accompanying decreased body weight. Although not intended as a weight loss agent, it is known to reduce weight by 1–2 kg alongside a low-calorie diet and its safety in pregnancy is well studied [61].

Many obese men and women also self-medicate with herbal supplements although their safety and effectiveness have not been demonstrated.

Unfortunately, much like with lifestyle intervention and behavior modification strategies, weight loss is modest at best, and dropout rates with these medications due to time and also side effects typically exceed 30% [76].

5.3 Bariatric surgery

There is an increasing number of bariatric surgical procedures being performed worldwide with nearly 200,000 cases being reported recently [77]. The surgeries vary between restrictive, such as the sleeve gastrectomy or the laparoscopic adjustable gastric banding and the malabsorptive procedures such as biliopancreatic diversion or a mixed restrictive/malabsorptive procedure such as the Roux en Y gastric bypass. Bariatric surgery is considered with morbid obesity (BMI > 40 kg/m^2) or with BMI > 35 kg/m^2 with concomitant medical conditions exacerbated by obesity [61].

The benefits of bariatric surgery include significant and long-term weight loss. The latest IFSO report demonstrated mean weight loss of 30% at 1 year postsurgery [77], and the Swedish Obese Study [61] showed significant weight reduction was maintained even after 10 years of follow-up [78]. Additionally, bariatric surgery has been shown to improve endocrine and metabolic profiles [61].

In women, bariatric surgery has been shown to improve menstrual regularity [79], correct ovulation [80], improve clinical and biochemical hyperandrogenism along with hyperinsulinemia and glycemic control, and improve both sexual function along with pregnancy rates [81–83].

In men, bariatric surgery improves hormone profiles by increasing testosterone and decreasing SHBG and estradiol [84]. Studies have not demonstrated an improvement in sperm quality, and in fact there have been case reports that have shown a deterioration on sperm parameters following surgery, likely due to nutritional deficiencies [48, 85]. This is in opposition to findings of longer-term stable sperm parameters following significant weight loss postbariatric surgery [86]. There is no doubt that more research needs to be done in this area to clarify this impact on male fertility.

The obstetric impact of bariatric surgery is profound with the risks of complications such as gestational diabetes, preeclampsia, and fetal macrosomia significantly reduced following surgery when compared to morbidly obese women [61]. Rare surgical complications (bowel obstruction, herniation, band events, and surgical line strictures) have been reported in pregnancy due to intra-abdominal pressure, displacement from the gravid uterus, and even hyperemesis [87, 88]. However, nutritional deficiencies due to malabsorptive-type surgery or noncompliance with long-term supplementation can have a significant effect on fertility and pregnancy outcomes. Deficiencies in iron, vitamin A, vitamin D, vitamin B12, vitamin K, and calcium can lead to maternal complications (e.g., anemia, osteopenia) and fetal complications (e.g., congenital abnormalities) [87]. Although there are no randomized prospective trials addressing time to conception after bariatric surgery, it is suggested to delay pregnancy 1–2 years postsurgery to avoid fetal exposure to nutritional deficiencies from rapid maternal weight loss [87, 89–91]. A large age and BMI-matched cohort study has demonstrated that the chance of preterm birth and small-for-gestational age (SGA) singletons were greater in women with a history of bariatric surgery than in women without such surgery and that the risk of still birth or neonatal death was slightly higher in the bariatric surgery group as well [92]. The median time from surgery to conception was 1.1 years. There does not appear to be any significant differences in obstetric or perinatal outcomes when comparing the different bariatric surgery procedures [93].

There are, however, studies comparing pregnancies conceived less than 1 year after bariatric surgery to those conceived greater than 1 year after surgery and found no difference in bariatric complications, pregnancy related, or perinatal outcomes [93, 94]. Therefore, when considering advanced age of the woman, the benefits of postponing pregnancy must be balanced against the risk of declining fertility due to age [4, 61].

6. Conclusion

Obesity is increasing globally in men and women, and the negative impact of overweight and obesity on reproductive health, fertility, pregnancy outcomes, and also transgenerational health is significant. Obesity impairs both natural and assisted conception and has been found to affect endocrine function, oocyte and sperm quality, embryo quality, and also endometrial receptivity and implantation. Pregnancy and live birth rates are lower, and miscarriage rates are higher in the setting of obesity. The metabolic and reproductive health of the offspring is also negatively affected by both maternal and paternal obesity.

Preconceptional weight loss is recommended for all women seeking fertility treatment, firstly through counseling, lifestyle intervention, and behavior modification and then with adjunctive pharmacological agents or bariatric surgery, with a delay to conception of at least 1 year following this. Careful consideration of the benefits of delaying conception for weight loss must be balanced against the possibility of declining fertility due to advancing age of the couple.

Acknowledgements

Ms. Helen Adams, Librarian, King Edward Memorial Hospital for Women.

Conflicts of interest

None.

Author details

Tamara Hunter[1*] and Roger Hart[2]

1 King Edward Memorial Hospital and Fertility Specialists of Western Australia, Perth, Australia

2 Division of Obstetrics and Gynaecology, University of Western Australia and Fertility Specialists of Western Australia, Perth, Australia

*Address all correspondence to: tamarajhunter@westnet.com.au

References

[1] World Health Organisation. Obesity. 2018 [updated 2018]. Available from: http://www.who.int/topics/obesity/en/

[2] World Health Organisation. Obesity and overweight. 2018 [updated 2018-02-16]. Available from: http://www.who.int/news-room/fact-sheets/detail/obesity-and-overweight

[3] Zegers-Hochschild F, Adamson GD, de Mouzon J, Ishihara O, Mansour R, Nygren K, et al. International Committee for Monitoring Assisted Reproductive Technology (ICMART) and the World Health Organization (WHO) revised glossary of ART terminology. Fertility and Sterility. 2009;**92**(5):1520-1524

[4] Practice Committe of the American Society for Reproductive Medicine. Obesity and reproduction: A committee opinion. Fertility and Sterility. 2015;**104**(5):1116-1126

[5] Escobar-Morreale HF. Surgical management of metabolic dysfunction in PCOS. Steroids. 2012;**77**:312-316

[6] Broughton DE, Moley KH. Obesity and female infertility: Potential mediators of obesity's impact. Fertility and Sterility. 2017;**107**(4):840-847

[7] Jain A, Polotsky AJ, Rochester D, Berga SL, Loucks T, Zeitlian G, et al. Pulsitile luteinizing hormone amplitude and progesterone metabolite excretion are reduced in obese women. The Journal of Clinical Endocrinology and Metabolism. 2007;**92**:2468-2473

[8] Wise LA, Rothman KJ, Mikkelsen EM, Sorensen HT, Riis A, Hatch EE. An internet-based prospective study of body size and time-to-pregnancy. Human Reproduction. 2010;**25**:253-264

[9] Ramlau-Hansen CH, Thulstrup AM, Nohr EA, Bonde JP, Sorensen TI, Olsen J. Subfecundity in overweight and obese couples. Human Reproduction. 2007;**22**:1634-1637

[10] Gesink Law DC, Maclehose RF, Longnecker MP. Obesity and time to pregnancy. Human Reproduction. 2007;**22**:414-420

[11] van der Steeg JW, Steures P, Eijkemans MJ, Habbema JD, Hompes PG, Burggraaff JM, et al. Obesity affects spontaneous pregnancy chances in subfertile, ovulatory women. Human Reproduction. 2008;**23**:324-328

[12] Luke B, Brown MB, Stern JE, Missmer SA, Fujimoto VY, Leach R, et al. Female obesity adversely affects assisted reproductive technology (ART) pregnancy and live birth rates. Human Reproduction. 2011;**26**(1):245-252

[13] Jungheim ES, Schon SB, Schulte MB, DeUgarte DA, Fowler SA, Tuuli MG. IVF outcomes in obese donor oocyte recipients: A systematic review and meta-analysis. Human Reproduction. 2013;**28**(10):2720-2727

[14] Esinler I, Bozdag G, Yarali H. Impact of isolated obesity on ICSI outcome. Reproductive Biomedicine Online. 2008;**17**(4):583-587

[15] Souter I, Baltagi LM, Kuleta D, Meeker JD, Petrozza JC. Women, weight, and fertility: The effect of body mass index on the outcome of superovulation/intrauterine insemination cycles. Fertility and Sterility. 2011;**95**(3):1042-1047

[16] Shah DK, Missmer SA, Berry KF, Racowsky C, Ginsburg ES. Effect of obesity on oocyte and embryo quality in women undergoing in vitro fertilization. Obstetrics and Gynecology. 2011;**118**(1):63-70

[17] Moragianni VA, Jones SM, Ryley DA. The effect of body mass index on the outcomes of first assisted reproductive technology cycles. Fertility and Sterility. 2012;**98**(1):102-108

[18] Pinborg A, Gaarslev C, Hougaard CO, Nyboe Andersen A, Andersen PK, Boivin J, et al. Influence of female bodyweight on IVF outcome: A longitudinal multicentre cohort study of 487 infertile couples. Reproductive Biomedicine Online. 2011;**23**(4):490-499

[19] Luzzo KM, Wang Q, Purcell SH, Chi M, Jimenez PT, Grindler N, et al. High fat diet induced developmental defects in the mouse: Oocyte meiotic aneuploidy and fetal growth retardation/brain defects. PLoS One. 2012;**7**(11):e49217

[20] Lane M, Zander-Fox DL, Robker RL, McPherson NO. Peri-conception parental obesity, reproductive health, and transgenerational impacts. Trends in Endocrinology and Metabolism. 2015;**26**(2):84-90

[21] Wu LL, Dunning KR, Yang X, Russell DL, Lane M, Norman RJ, et al. High-fat diet causes lipotoxicity responses in cumulus-oocyte complexes and decreased fertilization rates. Endocrinology. 2010;**151**(11):5438-5445

[22] Igosheva N, Abramov AY, Poston L, Eckert JJ, Fleming TP, Duchen MR, et al. Maternal diet-induced obesity alters mitochondrial activity and redox status in mouse oocytes and zygotes. PLoS One. 2010;**5**(4):e10074

[23] Carrell DT, Jones KP, Peterson CM, Aoki V, Emery BR, Campbell BR. Body mass index is inversely related to intrafollicular HCG concentrations, embryo quality and IVF outcome. Reproductive Biomedicine Online. 2001;**3**(2):109-111

[24] Metwally M, Cutting R, Tipton A, Skull J, Ledger WL, Li TC. Effect of increased body mass index on oocyte and embryo quality in IVF patients. Reproductive Biomedicine Online. 2007;**15**:532-538

[25] Leary C, Leese HJ, Sturmey RG. Human embryos from overweight and obese women display phenotypic and metabolic abnormalities. Human Reproduction. 2015;**30**(1):122-132

[26] Jungheim ES, Macones GA, Odem RR, Patterson BW, Lanzendorf SE, Ratts VS, et al. Associations between free fatty acids, cumulus oocyte complex morphology and ovarian function during in vitro fertilization. Fertility and Sterility. 2011;**95**(6):1970-1974

[27] Magarinos MP, Sanchez-Margalet V, Kotler M, Calvo JC, Varone CL. Leptin promotes cell proliferation and survival of trophoblastic cells. Biology of Reproduction. 2007;**76**(2):203-210

[28] Fedorcsak P, Dale PO, Storeng R, Ertzeid G, Bjercke S, Oldereid N, et al. Impact of overweight and underweight on assisted reproduction treatment. Human Reproduction. 2004;**19**(11):2523-2528

[29] Spandorfer SD, Kump L, Goldschlag D, Brodkin T, Davis OK, Rosenwaks Z. Obesity and in vitro fertilization: Negative influences on outcome. The Journal of Reproductive Medicine. 2004;**49**(12):973-977

[30] Dechaud H, Anahory T, Reyftmann L, Loup V, Hamamah S, Hedon B. Obesity does not adversely affect results in patients who are undergoing in vitro fertilization and embryo transfer. European Journal of Obstetrics, Gynecology, and Reproductive Biology. 2006;**127**(1):88-93

[31] Bellver J, Ayllon Y, Ferrando M, Melo M, Goyri E, Pellicer A, et al. Female obesity impairs in vitro fertilization outcome without affecting

embryo quality. Fertility and Sterility. 2010;**93**(2):447-454

[32] Brewer CJ, Balen AH. The adverse effects of obesity on conception and implantation. Reproduction. 2010;**140**(3):347-364

[33] Bellver J, Martinez-Conejero JA, Labarta E, Alama P, Melo MA, Remohi J, et al. Endometrial gene expression in the window of implantation is altered in obese women especially in association with polycystic ovary syndrome. Fertility and Sterility. 2011;**95**(7):2335-2341. 41 e1-8

[34] Bellver J, Melo MA, Bosch E, Serra V, Remohi J, Pellicer A. Obesity and poor reproductive outcome: The potential role of the endometrium. Fertility and Sterility. 2007;**88**(2):446-451

[35] Alvarez C, Alonso-Muriel I, Garcia G, Crespo J, Bellver J, Simon C, et al. Implantation is apparently unaffected by the dopamine agonist cabergoline when administered to prevent ovarian hyperstimulation syndrome in women undergoing assisted reproduction treatment: A pilot study. Human Reproduction. 2007;**22**(12):3210-3214

[36] DeUgarte DA, DeUgarte CM, Sahakian V. Surrogate obesity negatively impacts pregnancy rates in third-party reproduction. Fertility and Sterility. 2010;**93**(3):1008-1010

[37] Wattanakumtornkul S, Damario MA, Stevens Hall SA, Thornhill AR, Tummon IS. Body mass index and uterine receptivity in the oocyte donation model. Fertility and Sterility. 2003;**80**(2):336-340

[38] Loveland JB, McClamrock HD, Malinow AM, Sharara FI. Increased body mass index has a deleterious effect on in vitro fertilization outcome. Journal of Assisted Reproduction and Genetics. 2001;**18**(7):382-386

[39] Wang JX, Davies MJ, Norman RJ. Obesity increases the risk of spontaneous abortion during infertility treatment. Obesity Research. 2002;**10**(6):551-554

[40] Rittenberg V, Seshadri S, Sunkara SK, Sobaleva S, Oteng-Ntim E, El-Toukhy T. Effect of body mass index on IVF treatment outcome: An updated systematic review and meta-analysis. Reproductive Biomedicine Online. 2011;**23**(4):421-439

[41] Donnino MW, Rittenberger JC, Gaieski D, Cocchi MN, Giberson B, Peberdy MA, et al. The development and implementation of cardiac arrest centers. Resuscitation. 2011;**82**(8):974-978

[42] Bellver J, Rossal LP, Bosch E, Zuniga A, Corona JT, Melendez F, et al. Obesity and the risk of spontaneous abortion after oocyte donation. Fertility and Sterility. 2003;**79**(5):1136-1140

[43] Bellver J, Albert C, Labarta E, Pellicer A. Early pregnancy loss in women stimulated with gonadotropin-releasing hormone antagonist protocols according to oral contraceptive pill pretreatment. Fertility and Sterility. 2007;**87**(5):1098-1101

[44] Metwally M, Ong KJ, Ledger WL, Li TC. Does high body mass index increase the risk of miscarriage after spontaneous and assisted conception? A meta-analysis of the evidence. Fertility and Sterility. 2008;**90**(3):714-726

[45] Metwally M, Saravelos SH, Ledger WL, Li TC. Body mass index and risk of miscarriage in women with recurrent miscarriage. Fertility and Sterility. 2010;**94**(1):290-295

[46] MacDonald AA, Herbison GP, Showell M, Farquhar CM. The impact of body mass index on semen parameters and reproductive hormones in human

males: A systematic review with meta-analysis. Human Reproduction Update. 2010;**16**(3):293-311

[47] McPherson NO, Lane M. Male obesity and subfertility, is it really about increased adiposity? Asian Journal of Andrology. 2015;**17**(3):450-458

[48] Sermondade N, Dupont C, Faure C, Boubaya M, Cedrin-Durnerin I, Chavatte-Palmer P, et al. Body mass index is not associated with sperm-zona pellucida binding ability in subfertile males. Asian Journal of Andrology. 2013;**15**(5):626-629

[49] Lewis SE, John Aitken R, Conner SJ, Iuliis GD, Evenson DP, Henkel R, et al. The impact of sperm DNA damage in assisted conception and beyond: Recent advances in diagnosis and treatment. Reproductive Biomedicine Online. 2013;**27**(4):325-337

[50] Zhao J, Zhai L, Liu Z, Wu S, Xu L. Leptin level and oxidative stress contribute to obesity-induced low testosterone in murine testicular tissue. Oxidative Medicine and Cellular Longevity. 2014;**2014**:190945

[51] Duale N, Steffensen IL, Andersen J, Brevik A, Brunborg G, Lindeman B. Impaired sperm chromatin integrity in obese mice. Andrology. 2014;**2**(2):234-243

[52] Palmer NO, Bakos HW, Owens JA, Setchell BP, Lane M. Diet and exercise in an obese mouse fed a high-fat diet improve metabolic health and reverse perturbed sperm function. American Journal of Physiology. Endocrinology and Metabolism. 2012;**302**(7):E768-E780

[53] Jia YF, Feng Q, Ge ZY, Guo Y, Zhou F, Zhang KS, et al. Obesity impairs male fertility through long-term effects on spermatogenesis. BMC Urology. 2018;**18**(1):42

[54] Tamler R. Diabetes, obesity, and erectile dysfunction. Gender Medicine. 2009;**6**(Suppl 1):4-16

[55] Loche E, Ozanne SE. Non-genetic transmission of obesity—It's in your epigenes. Trends in Endocrinology and Metabolism. 2016;**27**(6):349-350

[56] Huypens P, Sass S, Wu M, Dyckhoff D, Tschop M, Theis F, et al. Epigenetic germline inheritance of diet-induced obesity and insulin resistance. Nature Genetics. 2016;**48**(5):497-499

[57] Fullston T, Ohlsson Teague EM, Palmer NO, DeBlasio MJ, Mitchell M, Corbett M, et al. Paternal obesity initiates metabolic disturbances in two generations of mice with incomplete penetrance to the F2 generation and alters the transcriptional profile of testis and sperm microRNA content. The FASEB Journal. 2013;**27**(10):4226-4243

[58] Tunc O, Tremellen K. Oxidative DNA damage impairs global sperm DNA methylation in infertile men. Journal of Assisted Reproduction and Genetics. 2009;**26**(9-10):537-544

[59] Chen Q, Yan M, Cao Z, Li X, Zhang Y, Shi J, et al. Sperm tsRNAs contribute to intergenerational inheritance of an acquired metabolic disorder. Science. 2016;**351**(6271):397-400

[60] Soubry A, Murphy SK, Wang F, Huang Z, Vidal AC, Fuemmeler BF, et al. Newborns of obese parents have altered DNA methylation patterns at imprinted genes. International Journal of Obesity. 2015;**39**(4):650-657

[61] Mahutte N, Kamga-Ngande C, Sharma A, Sylvestre C. Obesity and reproduction. Journal of Obstetrics and Gynaecology Canada. 2018;**40**(7):950-966

[62] Legro RS, Dodson WC, Kunselman AR, Stetter CM, Kris-Etherton PM, Williams NI, et al. Benefit of delayed

fertility therapy with preconception weight loss over immediate therapy in obese women with PCOS. The Journal of Clinical Endocrinology and Metabolism. 2016;**101**(7):2658-2666

[63] Espinos JJ, Polo A, Sanchez-Hernandez J, Bordas R, Pares P, Martinez O, et al. Weight decrease improves live birth rates in obese women undergoing IVF: A pilot study. Reproductive Biomedicine Online. 2017;**35**(4):417-424

[64] Clark AM, Thornley B, Tomlinson L, Galletley C, Norman RJ. Weight loss in obese infertile women results in improvement in reproductive outcome for all forms of fertility treatment. Human Reproduction. 1998;**13**(6):1502-1505

[65] Einarsson S, Bergh C, Friberg B, Pinborg A, Klajnbard A, Karlstrom PO, et al. Weight reduction intervention for obese infertile women prior to IVF: A randomized controlled trial. Human Reproduction. 2017;**32**(8):1621-1630

[66] Tuomilehto J, Lindstrom J, Eriksson JG, Valle TT, Hamalainen H, Ilanne-Parikka P, et al. Prevention of type 2 diabetes mellitus by changes in lifestyle among subjects with impaired glucose tolerance. The New England Journal of Medicine. 2001;**344**(18):1343-1350

[67] Wing RR, Hill JO. Successful weight loss maintenance. Annual Review of Nutrition. 2001;**21**:323-341

[68] Palomba S, Falbo A, Valli B, Morini D, Villani MT, Nicoli A, et al. Physical activity before IVF and ICSI cycles in infertile obese women: An observational cohort study. Reproductive Biomedicine Online. 2014;**29**(1):72-79

[69] Meldrum DR. Introduction: Obesity and reproduction. Fertility and Sterility. 2017;**107**(4):831-832

[70] Li Z, Maglione M, Tu W, Mojica W, Arterburn D, Shugarman LR, et al. Meta-analysis: Pharmacologic treatment of obesity. Annals of Internal Medicine. 2005;**142**(7):532-546

[71] Apovian CM, Aronne LJ, Bessesen DH, McDonnell ME, Murad MH, Pagotto U, et al. Pharmacological management of obesity: An endocrine society clinical practice guideline. The Journal of Clinical Endocrinology and Metabolism. 2015;**100**(2):342-362

[72] Lee PC, Dixon J. Pharmacotherapy for obesity. Australian Family Physician. 2017;**46**(7):472-477

[73] Pi-Sunyer X, Astrup A, Fujioka K, Greenway F, Halpern A, Krempf M, et al. A randomized, controlled trial of 3.0 mg of liraglutide in weight management. The New England Journal of Medicine. 2015;**373**(1):11-22

[74] Greenway FL, Fujioka K, Plodkowski RA, Mudaliar S, Guttadauria M, Erickson J, et al. Effect of naltrexone plus bupropion on weight loss in overweight and obese adults (COR-I): A multicentre, randomised, double-blind, placebo-controlled, phase 3 trial. Lancet. 2010;**376**(9741):595-605

[75] Smith SR, Weissman NJ, Anderson CM, Sanchez M, Chuang E, Stubbe S, et al. Multicenter, placebo-controlled trial of lorcaserin for weight management. The New England Journal of Medicine. 2010;**363**(3):245-256

[76] Fabricatore AN, Wadden TA, Moore RH, Butryn ML, Gravallese EA, Erondu NE, et al. Attrition from randomized controlled trials of pharmacological weight loss agents: A systematic review and analysis. Obesity Reviews. 2009;**10**(3):333-341

[77] Higa K, Himpens J, Welbourn R, Dixon J, Kinsman R, Walton P. Third IFSO Global Registry Report 2017.

Updated August 2017. Available from: http://www.ifso.com/wp-content/themes/ypo-theme/pdfs/final-3rd-ifso-report-21st-august-2017.pdf

[78] Sjostrom L, Lindroos AK, Peltonen M, Torgerson J, Bouchard C, Carlsson B, et al. Lifestyle, diabetes, and cardiovascular risk factors 10 years after bariatric surgery. The New England Journal of Medicine. 2004;**351**(26):2683-2693

[79] Teitelman M, Grotegut CA, Williams NN, Lewis JD. The impact of bariatric surgery on menstrual patterns. Obesity Surgery. 2006;**16**(11):1457-1463

[80] Tan O, Carr BR. The impact of bariatric surgery on obesity-related infertility and in vitro fertilization outcomes. Seminars in Reproductive Medicine. 2012;**30**(6):517-528

[81] Legro RS, Dodson WC, Gnatuk CL, Estes SJ, Kunselman AR, Meadows JW, et al. Effects of gastric bypass surgery on female reproductive function. The Journal of Clinical Endocrinology and Metabolism. 2012;**97**(12):4540-4548

[82] Marceau P, Kaufman D, Biron S, Hould FS, Lebel S, Marceau S, et al. Outcome of pregnancies after biliopancreatic diversion. Obesity Surgery. 2004;**14**(3):318-324

[83] Musella M, Milone M, Bellini M, Sosa Fernandez LM, Leongito M, Milone F. Effect of bariatric surgery on obesity-related infertility. Surgery for Obesity and Related Diseases. 2012;**8**(4):445-449

[84] Reis LO, Zani EL, Saad RD, Chaim EA, de Oliveira LC, Fregonesi A. Bariatric surgery does not interfere with sperm quality—A preliminary long-term study. Reproductive Sciences. 2012;**19**(10):1057-1062

[85] di Frega AS, Dale B, Di Matteo L, Wilding M. Secondary male factor infertility after Roux-en-Y gastric bypass for morbid obesity: Case report. Human Reproduction. 2005;**20**(4):997-998

[86] Legro RS, Kunselman AR, Meadows JW, Kesner JS, Krieg EF, Rogers AM, et al. Time-related increase in urinary testosterone levels and stable semen analysis parameters after bariatric surgery in men. Reproductive Biomedicine Online. 2015;**30**(2):150-156

[87] Guelinckx I, Devlieger R, Vansant G. Reproductive outcome after bariatric surgery: A critical review. Human Reproduction Update. 2009;**15**(2):189-201

[88] Hezelgrave NL, Oteng-Ntim E. Pregnancy after bariatric surgery: A review. Journal of Obesity. 2011;**2011**:501939

[89] Beard JH, Bell RL, Duffy AJ. Reproductive considerations and pregnancy after bariatric surgery: Current evidence and recommendations. Obesity Surgery. 2008;**18**(8):1023-1027

[90] Monson M, Jackson M. Pregnancy after bariatric surgery. Clinical Obstetrics and Gynecology. 2016;**59**(1):158-171

[91] American Dietetic A, American Society of N, Siega-Riz AM, King JC. Position of the American Dietetic Association and American Society for Nutrition: Obesity, reproduction, and pregnancy outcomes. Journal of the American Dietetic Association. 2009;**109**(5):918-927

[92] Johansson K, Cnattingius S, Naslund I, Roos N, Trolle Lagerros Y, Granath F, et al. Outcomes of pregnancy after bariatric surgery. The New England Journal of Medicine. 2015;**372**(9):814-824

[93] Sheiner E, Balaban E, Dreiher J, Levi I, Levy A. Pregnancy outcome in patients following different types of bariatric surgeries. Obesity Surgery. 2009;**19**(9):1286-1292

[94] Kjaer MM, Nilas L. Timing of pregnancy after gastric bypass-a national register-based cohort study. Obesity Surgery. 2013;**23**(8):1281-1285

Chapter 5

Treatment Options in Morbid Obesity

Tülay Diken Allahverdi

Abstract

Obesity has become the most common fatal and the second most common preventable epidemic disease after smoking in the world. Although it causes many morbidities, the psychosocial challenges it creates in the patients and the huge financial burden for its treatment are the main problems. Medical treatment for weight loss is usually inadequate, and surgery has become a major part of morbid obesity treatment. Roux-en-Y gastric bypass (RYGB), sleeve gastrectomy (SG), adjustable gastric band (AGB), and biliopancreatic diversion (BPD) are the most common current surgical procedures, and all can be performed laparoscopically. Eating less and early satiety due to the reduction of gastric volume with surgery and the disruption of absorption as a result of the bypass lead to significant weight loss.

Keywords: morbid obesity, surgical treatment, laparoscopy

1. Introduction

Obesity is a chronic disease and is the result of the energy obtained from food being higher than the energy consumed and is characterized by an increase in the body's fat mass compared to the lean mass. Obesity is an important health problem that can cause various problems and even death by affecting all organs and systems of the body and especially the cardiovascular and endocrine systems. Obesity is accepted as one of the ten most risky diseases by the World Health Organization (WHO), which has also found it to be closely associated with cancer in recent studies. The prevalence of obesity and being overweight has been increasing in many industrial countries and is now creating a difficult problem for many populations [1]. There has been no other problem affecting humanity that is as common as obesity. Obesity develops by a mechanism that depends on many factors such as eating habits, toxic chemicals, and lifestyle unlike diseases caused by an infectious agent such as the plague, tuberculosis, or AIDS. What this mechanism is or whether obesity is really a disease is not yet clear.

The surgical treatment of obesity is named bariatric surgery. Long-term permanent weight loss is provided, many comorbid diseases are prevented, and survival is increased by decreasing the metabolic effects of obesity as a result of bariatric surgery. Sustainable weight loss can only be achieved by bariatric surgery, and it decreases the excess weight by 50% [2]. Patients scheduled to undergo surgery should be clearly informed on the expected benefit, risk and long-term outcomes of surgery, and the requirement for lifelong nutritional counseling and biochemical follow-up.

1.1 Bariatric surgery indications

- BMI >40 kg/m^2 or the presence of additional disease (type 2 diabetes, hypertension, sleep apnea, hyperlipidemia) together with BMI >35 kg/m^2
- Acceptable surgical risk
- Unsuccessful nonsurgical treatments
- Being psychologically stable and lack of alcohol or drug addiction
- The patient being well motivated and being informed about the surgery and its sequelae
- Lack of medical problems that will prevent the increased life expectation as a result of the surgery
- Lack of uncontrolled psychotic and depressive disorders
- Presence of full family and social support

1.2 The most commonly performed bariatric surgical procedures

- Restrictive procedures
- Laparoscopic adjustable gastric band (LAGB)
- Sleeve gastrectomy (SG)
- Vertical banded gastroplasty (VBG)
- Absorption-disrupting procedures
- Biliopancreatic diversion (BPD)
- Jejunoileal bypass (JIB)
- Combined restrictive and absorption-disruptive procedures
- Roux-en-Y gastric bypass (RYGB)
- Duodenal switch (DS) along with BPD

The mechanism of action of bariatric surgical procedures is related to the complex interactions between gastric resection and malabsorption as well as the hormonal and neural signals affecting hunger and satiety. Buchwald et al. [3] reported the rate of improvement in diabetes with bariatric surgery as 56.7, 79.7, 80.3, and 95.1% following adjustable gastric band (AGB), Roux-en-Y gastric bypass, and biliopancreatic diversion with duodenal switch (BPD-DS), respectively, in a meta-analysis. Complete diabetes remission was observed in 78% of the patients. The lipid profile is also improved in 70% of the patients after bariatric surgery. The total cholesterol, LDL, and triglyceride levels are decreased, but no significant change has been reported for HDL levels.

Mortality rates in bariatric surgical procedures are equal to those observed with small intra-abdominal operations such as laparoscopic cholecystectomy (0.3–0.6%) [4].

2. Laparoscopic Roux-en-Y gastric bypass (LRYGB)

LRYGB is the most commonly used restrictive method. It is reported to be the gold standard in the surgical treatment of morbid obesity as it provides long-term weight loss and has acceptable morbidity and mortality [5]. The gastric bypass method in bariatric surgery was first suggested by Edward E. Mason [6]. While 90% of the stomach volume is reduced, malabsorption is ensured by bypassing the duodenum in this method. The main aim is to create a proximal small-volume (<20 ml) gastric pouch that is completely detached from the stomach (**Figure 1**). The Roux limb can be pulled up from the front of the colon and stomach, from the front of the colon and the back of the stomach, or from the back of the colon and stomach for gastrojejunostomy. Transoral circular stapling, linear stapling, manual suturing, or transgastric circular stapling can be used for gastrojejunostomy. The biliopancreatic limb is prepared at a length of 50 cm and the Roux limb at a length of 100–150 cm distal to the Treitz ligament. Once the stomach is cut perpendicularly to the small curvature and 3–5 cm distal to the esophagogastric junction with a linear stapler (60 mm long and 3.8 mm thick), the pouch is formed by completing the cutting action toward the angle of His. Postoperative fluid support and ensuring adequate urine output are very important. The results and any nutritional deficiency should be checked at the postoperative third week, the third and sixth months, and the first year [7]. These patients lose 60–80% of their extra weight within 1 year after the surgery. Consequently, a significant improvement is seen in

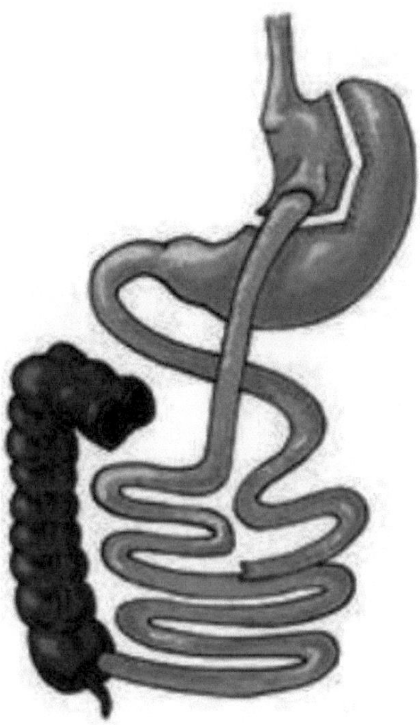

Figure 1.
Roux-en-Y gastric bypass.

the comorbid diseases. Mortality is <1% and morbidity is 15%. Complications such as postoperative leakage (1–2%), stenosis (1–19%), small bowel obstruction-internal hernia (7%), and marginal ulcer (3–15%) can be seen. Urgent surgical intervention is required when intestinal obstruction is suspected as it may cause long segment necrosis. Roux-en-Y gastric bypass is more effective than a laparoscopic adjustable gastric band especially in the treatment of type 2 DM and gastroesophageal reflux disease (GERD) symptoms.

3. Sleeve gastrectomy (vertical gastrectomy)

Sleeve gastrectomy was first introduced as a restrictive component of duodenal switch surgery. Adequate weight loss at an early period is seen with sleeve gastrectomy alone in patients who are very obese and at risk with duodenal switch (DS) surgery [8, 9]. This method has been put into practice as a risk-reducing method in patients who cannot tolerate high-risk and long-term procedures [9]. Laparoscopic sleeve gastrectomy (LSG) has become a safe and efficient primary bariatric surgical method with increasing frequency of use and high popularity for both surgeons and patients [2]. Laparoscopic sleeve gastrectomy constitutes 5% of all bariatric surgical procedures, and the number of patients is increasing rapidly [10]. A narrow tubular stomach is created with this method (**Figure 2**). Stomach resection is performed after releasing the large curvatura pylori 2–3 cm proximal to His angle. A tissue stapler 4.5 mm in size (thick) is used in the antrum and 3.8 mm in size (medium) for the other parts of the stomach. To avoid leaving a large fundus pouch, meticulous posterior dissection should be performed so that the His angle is visible. If the lateral traction of the stomach is not good, a spiral-shaped resection line may develop. To decrease the risk of leakage, 1 cm of gastric serosa should be seen on the left side of the stapler cartridge before firing the final stapler. After resection, leakage and hemorrhage in the stapler line is checked with the endoscope. In the case of possible leakage, the omentum is sutured to the suture line in order to create a potential barrier. The sleeve tube is fixed and bending of the stomach from the incisura angularis is prevented by suturing the omentum or gastrocolic fat [11–13].

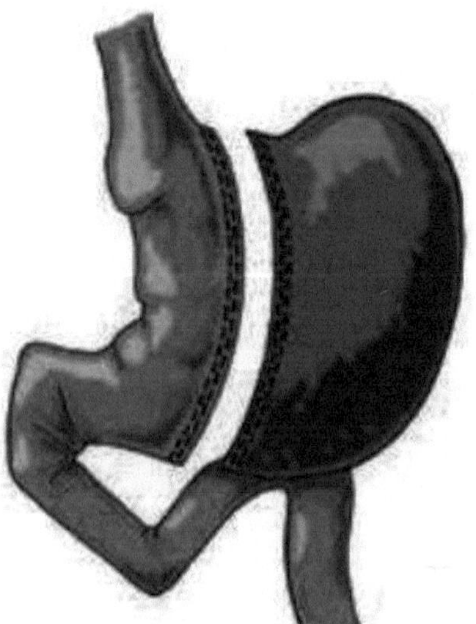

Figure 2.
Sleeve gastrectomy.

Laparoscopic sleeve gastrectomy is preferred in the super obese and in patients who have a BMI of <50 kg/m^2 and want to undergo surgery with this method. Mean loss in excess weight was reported as 55% with a complication rate of 8% and mortality rate of 0.19% in the review of 2500 patients (mean BMI: 51.2 kg/m^2) where this method had been preferred [9]. While the diabetes remission rate following laparoscopic sleeve gastrectomy is reported to be 66.2%, a new bariatric procedure may be required later on in 15% of the patients [9]. Laparoscopic sleeve gastrectomy has become a commonly preferred method by itself or combined with other methods in the treatment of morbid obesity [14]. The most important complication is leakage (2%) and is often seen near the angle of His. Placing the end of the stapler line close to the esophagus, stenosis of the incisura angularis and bending of the tubular stomach are among the causes of leakage. Gastroesophageal reflux occurs in 26% of the patients after laparoscopic sleeve gastrectomy [7]. Revision surgery should be performed in the case of treatment-resistant gastroesophageal reflux.

4. Laparoscopic adjustable gastric band

The laparoscopic adjustable gastric band method has been available in the USA since 2001 [15]. This method decreases the food intake with its complete restrictive effect and results in loss of weight. An inflatable silicone band is wrapped around the stomach 3 cm below the esophagogastric junction, and a reservoir of 25–30 cm long is formed at the proximal section. At the other end of the band, there is a subcutaneously placed port (**Figure 3**). The calibration of the gastric opening can be changed by fluoroscopy-guided filling and emptying of the silicone band. The band is initially inserted in completely deflated form. The pars flaccida technique has become the standard since band prolapse and erosion are less common in this way. The laparoscopic adjustable gastric band method requires frequent follow-up and should therefore only be performed in patients who live in close proximity to the hospital. Only multivitamins are recommended after the surgery. Adjustment of the band is as important as the surgery itself, and weight loss of 0.5 kg per week is ideal with this method [16]. Patients lose 58–60% of their extra weight in 7–8 years after

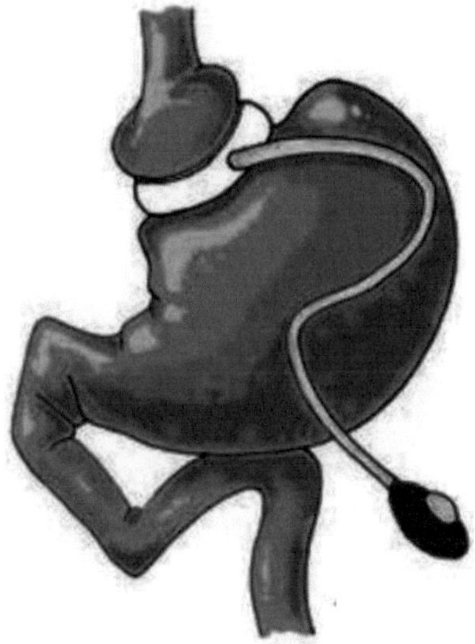

Figure 3.
Laparoscopic adjustable gastric band.

the surgery. The complication and mortality rate are less than the absorption-disrupting techniques [7]. Prolapse (3%), displacement (<3%), band erosion (1–2%), and port and tube complications (5%) can be seen. Although a high reoperation ratio is the major disadvantage, the technique is still popular in the USA [17].

5. Biliopancreatic diversion with duodenal switch

The biliopancreatic diversion with duodenal switch (BPDDS) procedure is often referred to as DS surgery. This technique is a modification of the original biliopancreatic diversion defined by Scapinaro et al. [18, 19] in 1979. The three main components of this technique are pylor-protected gastric tube formation, distal ileoileal anastomosis, and proximal duodenoileal anastomosis (**Figure 4**). Three intestinal limbs are formed in this method. Food passes through one limb (Roux limb), the fluid of the digestive organs (bile) from one limb (biliopancreatic limb), and food and digestive fluids from the common limb. While the small curvature of the stomach is removed and the pylor is preserved in biliopancreatic diversion with duodenal switch surgery, the pylor was also removed by distal gastric resection in the original surgery of Scapinaro. The gastric pouch is 250 ml in size, and malabsorption is created by Roux-en-Y reconstruction of the distal intestines in both techniques. The main limb length is 50–100 cm and the alimentary limb 250 cm, and the biliopancreatic limb is connected to a location 100 cm proximal to the ileocecal valve. Since the pylor is preserved in the biliopancreatic diversion with duodenal switch technique, complications such as loop formation, dumping, and marginal ulcers are less common. The method can also be performed in stages to reduce complications. If adequate weight loss cannot be provided with laparoscopic sleeve gastrectomy, the biliopancreatic diversion with duodenal switch procedure is performed 6–12 months later. Glucose control in severely obese patients with type 2 diabetes is better with biliopancreatic diversion with duodenal switch surgery than medical treatment. Although the technique is well described and provides effective weight loss, biliopancreatic diversion with duodenal switch procedure is not commonly used. While early weight loss is provided by the sleeve gastrectomy, impaired fat absorption is responsible for the long-term weight loss. The decrease in ghrelin and increase in peptide YY after the biliopancreatic diversion with duodenal

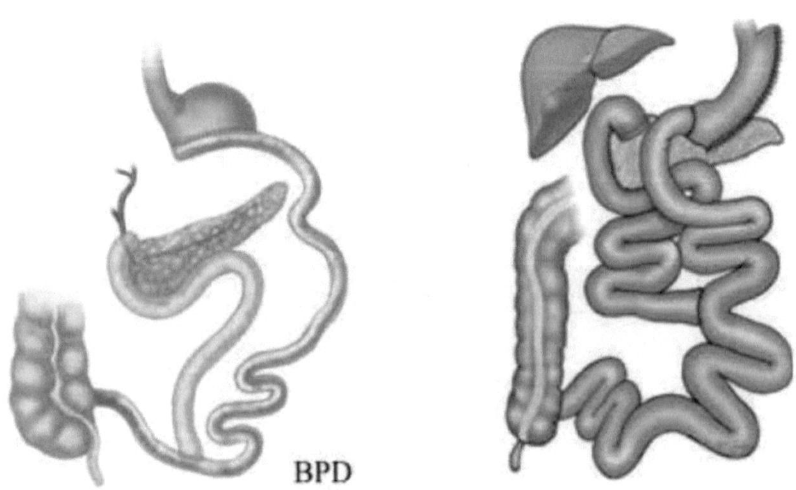

Figure 4.
Biliopancreatic diversion and duodenal switch.

switch procedure also increase weight loss. Mechanical changes as well as hormonal changes may therefore be responsible for the weight loss in this technique [20]. The surgical mortality rate is around 1%. The patients require high doses of vitamin and mineral supplementation after the surgery. There is significant improvement in the comorbid conditions after biliopancreatic diversion with duodenal switch. While 92% of diabetics and 90% of those with sleep apnea show full resolution, 80% of asthmatics decrease the dose of their medication [21, 22]. Close follow-up and vitamin supplements are necessary to prevent postoperative malnutrition. This method can be recommended as a revision method for severely obese patients, those who cannot exercise and stick to a diet after restrictive methods, and after any previous unsuccessful surgeries. This method should not be performed in those who cannot be monitored closely, who do not have adequate income for vitamin support, and previously suffered from calcium, iron, vitamin, and mineral deficiencies.

Vertical banded gastroplasty, laparoscopic mini-gastric bypass (LMGB), and laparoscopic large curvature plication (LLCP) are methods that are rarely used in morbid obesity surgery.

Author details

Tülay Diken Allahverdi
University of Kafkas, School of Medicine, Department of General Surgery, Kars, Turkey

*Address all correspondence to: drtulaydiken@hotmail.com

References

[1] Prevention and Management of the Global Epidemic of Obesity. Report of the WHO Consultation on Obesity; Geneva; June 3-5, 1997

[2] Brethauer SA. Sleeve gastrectomy. Surgical Clinics of North America. 2011;**91**:1265-1279. DOI: 10.1016/j.suc.2011.08.012

[3] Dixon JB, Zimmet P, Alberti KG, Rubino F. Bariatric surgery: An IDF statement for obese type 2 diabetes. Diabetic Medicine. 2011;**28**:628-642

[4] Khuri SF, Najjar SF, Daley J, VA National Surgical Quality Improvement Program, et al. Comparison of surgical outcomes between teaching and non-teaching hospitals in the Department of Veterans Affairs. Annals of Surgery. 2001;**234**:370-382. DOI: 10.1097/00000658-200109000-00011

[5] Wittgrove AC, Clark GW. Laparoscopic gastric bypass, Roux-en-Y-500 patients: Technique and results, with 3-60 month follow-up. Obesity Surgery. 2000;**10**:233-239. DOI: 10.1381/096089200321643511

[6] Powell M, Fernandez AZ. Surgical treatment for morbid obesity: The laparoscopic Roux-en-Y gastric bypass. Surgical Clinics of North America. 2011;**91**:1203-1224. DOI: 10.1016/j.suc.2011.08.0133

[7] Schirmer B, Schauer PR. The surgical management of obesity. In: Schwartz's Principles of Surgery. 2010. pp. 949-978

[8] Mason EE, Ito C. Gastric bypass in obesity. The Surgical Clinics of North America. 1967;**47**:1345-1351

[9] Brethauer SA, Hammel JP, Schauer PR. Systematic review of sleeve gastrectomy as staging and primary bariatric procedure. Surgery for Obesity and Related Diseases. 2009;**5**:469-475. DOI: 10.1016/j.soard.2009.05.011

[10] Regan JP, Inabnet WB, Gagner M, et al. Early experience with two-stage laparoscopic Roux-en-Y gastric bypass as an alternative in the super-super obese patient. Obesity Surgery. 2003;**13**:861-864

[11] Buchwald H, Oien DM. Metabolic/bariatric surgery worldwide 2008. Obesity Surgery. 2009;**19**:1605-1611. DOI: 10.1007/s11695-009-0014-5

[12] Karamanakos SN, Vagenas K, Kalfarentzos F, et al. Weight loss, appetite suppression, and changes in fasting and postprandial ghrelin and peptide-YY levels after Roux-en-Y gastric bypass and sleeve gastrectomy: A prospective, double blind study. Annals of Surgery. 2008;**247**:401-407. DOI: 10.1097/SLA.0b013e318156f012

[13] Melissas J, Daskalakis M, Koukouraki S, et al. Sleeve gastrectomy—A "food limiting" operation. Obesity Surgery. 2008;**18**:1251-1256. DOI: 10.1007/s11695-008-9634-4 22

[14] Gill RS, Birch DW, Shi X, et al. Sleeve gastrectomy and type 2 diabetes mellitus: A systematic review. Surgery for Obesity and Related Diseases. 2010;**6**:707-713

[15] Bohdjalian A, Langer FB, Shakeri-Leidenmuhler S, et al. Sleeve gastrectomy as sole and definitive bariatric procedure: 5-year results for weight loss and ghrelin. Obesity Surgery. 2010;**20**:535-540. DOI: 10.1007/s11695-009-0066-6

[16] Himpens J, Dobbeleir J, Peeters G. Long-term results of laparoscopic sleeve gastrectomy for obesity. Annals of Surgery. 2010;**252**:319-249. DOI: 10.1097/SLA.0b013e3181e90b31

[17] McBride CL, Vishal K. Evolution of laparoscopic adjustable gastric banding. Surgical Clinics of North America. 2011;**91**:1239-1247. DOI: 10.1016/j.suc.2011.08.006

[18] Freeman L, Brown WA, Korin A, et al. An approach to the assessment and management of the laparoscopic adjustable gastric band patient in the emergency department. Emergency Medicine Australasia. 2011;**23**:186-194

[19] Scopinaro N, Gianetta E, Civalleri D, et al. Biliopancreatic bypass for obesity: II. Initial experience in man. The British Journal of Surgery. 1979;**66**:618-620. DOI: 10.1002/bjs.1800660906

[20] Sudan R, Jacobs DO. Biliopancreatic diversion with duodenal switch. Surgical Clinics of North America. 2011;**91**:1281-1293. DOI: 10.1016/j.suc.2011.08.015 30

[21] Marceau P, Biron S, Hould FS, et al. Duodenal switch improved standard biliopancreatic diversion: A retrospective study. Surgery for Obesity and Related Diseases. 2009;**5**:43-47. DOI: 10.1016/j.soard.2008.03.244

[22] Prachand VN, Ward M, Alverdy JC. Duodenal switch provides superior resolution of metabolic comorbidities independent of weight loss in the super-obese (BMI > or = 50 kg/m^2) compared with gastric bypass. Journal of Gastrointestinal Surgery. 2010;**14**:211-220. DOI: 10.1007/s11605-009-1101-6